About the author and photographer

In 1975, Governor-General Jules Leger presented the Michener Award for meritorious public service through journalism to George Hutchison and Dick Wallace, in recognition of the coverage given by the London *Free Press* to the mercury crisis in Ontario.

George Hutchison, a native of Toronto, joined the London *Free Press* in 1964. In 1972 he received a National Newspaper Award for feature writing and an NNA merit citation for spot news reporting. That year he also won a Canada-wide conservation writing competition for the F. H. Kortright award.

Hutchison has just completed a year of study at the University of Toronto as a Southam fellow.

Dick Wallace has been with the London *Free Press* for twenty years and his work has appeared in several magazines, including *Weekend, Saturday Night, People,* and *Editor and Publisher.* In 1966, he won a national competition sponsored by the Professional Photographers of Canada . His photographs have been exhibited in The Hague (the Netherlands), Winnipeg, Montreal and in his native London.

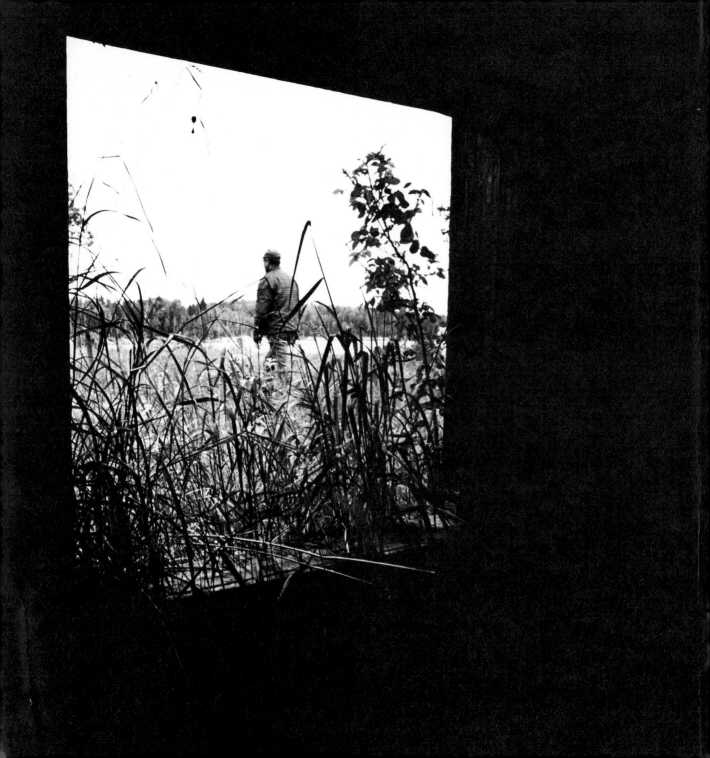

Grassy Narrows

Text by George Hutchison
Photos by Dick Wallace

Foreword by Philippe Cousteau

Van Nostrand Reinhold Ltd., *Toronto*
New York   Cincinnati   London   Melbourne

ISBN 0 442 29877 3
Library of Congress Number 77-72973

Design by Brant Cowie/Artplus
Maps by Julian Cleva

Printed and bound in Canada by The Hunter Rose Company
77 78 79 80 81 82 83 8 7 6 5 4 3 2 1

Canadian Cataloguing in Publication Data

Hutchison, George, 1940-
    Grassy Narrows

ISBN 0-442-29877-3 pa.

1. Water — Pollution — Economic aspects — Ontario. 2. Water — Pollution — Environmental aspects — Ontario. 3. Mercury — Toxicology. 4. Grassy Narrows, Ont. (Indian reserve) I. Wallace, Dick, 1938-   II. Title.

TD427.M4H8   363.6'1'097131   C77-001216-7

Photograph Credits

All the photographs in this book are by Dick Wallace; however, the following are copyright© 1975 by the London *Free Press* and are used with their permission: cover, 23, 28, 29, 30, 57, 59, 71, 79, 86, 87, 89, 115, 121, 122, 123, 124, 126, 127, 128, 129, 130.

Frontispiece: At the old village of Grassy Narrows, 1976.

Acknowledgment

Many people have made this book possible. We thank the management and staff of the London *Free Press* for its support and dedication to the story: Walter Blackburn, Peter White, Bill Heine, Jack Briglia, Jim O'Neail, Jack Burnett; Edythe Cusack and her library staff; Del Bell, Neil Morris, Cheryl Hamilton and Derek Hodgson.

Government officials and politicians have given of their time. The president of Reed Paper Company, the critical industry in this piece, agreed to be interviewed. His answers may not always satisfy the reader, but they are here and lend a perspective which might otherwise have been lost.

Our families — Elaine, Tracey, Blake, Chris and Natasha — willingly reorganized their lives around our disruptive schedules, thereby assuming an equal share in the responsibility for getting the job done.

Al Dickie, Dave Allen, Brian Vallee, Charlotte Montgomery, Harold Greer and Norm Webster, all members of the Queen's Park press gallery, contributed by their unselfish assistance.

The author wrote much of this book while attending the University of Toronto on a fellowship provided by the Southam Press Ltd. We extend our gratitude to the company and to two colleagues at Massey College, Kathy Brooks of the *Toronto Sun* and and Dr. Bernard von Graeve of Trent University. We also wish to thank Dr. Carlton Williams, retiring president of the University of Western

Ontario, Mrs. Win Miller of the Chatham bureau of the London *Free Press,* Dr. Norvald Fimreite of the University of Tromso, Norway, Dr. Ross Hume Hall, of McMaster University, Hamilton, Dr. Mario Faveri of the London office of the Addiction Research Foundation, and Ingrid Cook, Trade Editor at Van Nostrand Reinhold.

The Lake St. Clair fishermen have been cordial and co-operative; special thanks to Dime Jubenville and Lawrence Drouillard.

Our trip to Japan gave this project a deeper meaning. Our thanks are extended to Aileen Smith, who served as interpreter and guide, and her husband Gene, whom we have yet to meet beyond his award-winning photography. Their book on the Minamata tragedy has inspired us to make our own efforts at documenting the effects of mercury on an unsuspecting community. Thanks also to doctors Tadao Takeuchi, Masazumi Harada and Jun Ui. Tsuginori Hamamoto, chairman of the Minamata Disease Patients' Alliance, and Teruo Kawamoto, a fearless fighter in the long struggle for justice, were articulate spokesmen for the victims of Minamata Disease. Patients and families exposed to us the depths of their personal tragedies.

In the northwest, we received valuable assistance from Dr. Peter Newberry, the Quaker physician working at Grassy Narrows, Jill Torrie, a field worker with the National Indian Brotherhood, and Dennis Clark, the principal of the Grassy Narrows School. Barney Lamm and his wife Marion co-operated with us to take pollution beyond the abstract. Barney Lamm is a rich man with a cause; his interests are financial as well as moral. He co-operated fully with us, but he neither suggested nor commissioned the writing of this book, nor did he invest financially in it, contrary to rumors which have been heard in the north and voiced by industry.

None have given more than the people of Grassy Narrows. They allowed us into their homes and their lives. We pray that their trust has been rewarded.

G.H.
D.W.

To Andy Keewatin, Bill Fobister, Sharon Fobister, Tommy Keesick, Gabe Kokohopenace, Marcel and Rosy Pahpasay, Joe Quoquat, Joe Loon and all the people of Grassy Narrows.

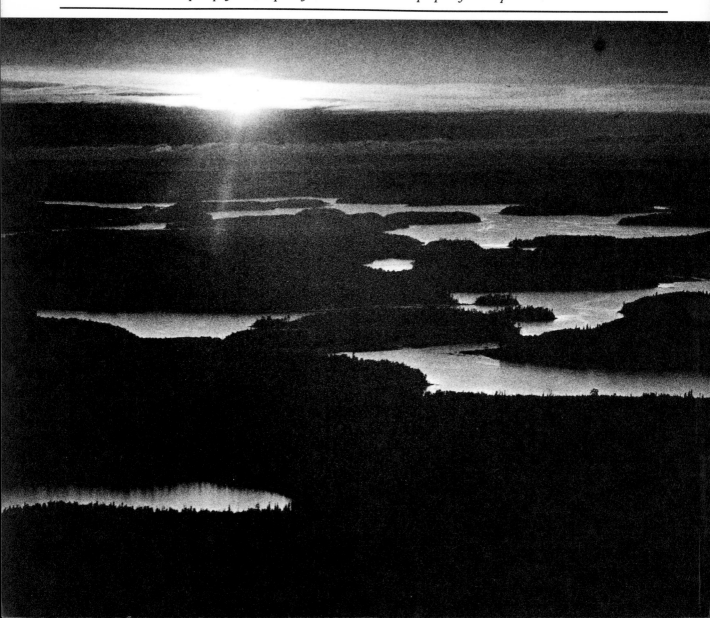

Contents

Foreword

When anger and emotion well in your heart beyond the bearable, frustration and puzzlement paralyze your chest, your field of vision narrows and you choke on uncertain words, it is the *crève-coeur*.*

It is the *crève-coeur* when, as happened in Minamata, Japan, executives in charge, in their air-conditioned offices, shrug their shoulders with apparent sorrow, and let pollution kill hundreds of people because to save them is not "economically feasible." It is also when, as happened in Italy, the faces of children swell into disgusting masks and that the horror is explained and justified by financial excuses: the system that could have prevented the deadly gas from leaking was too expensive. When Chief Mandamin of the White Dog reserve told me with a humor loaded by 300 years of history, "Maybe they found a new way to get rid of us Indians," that too is the *crève-coeur*. And all the compassionate and reassuring words die somewhere within oneself smothered by shame and anger.

Because those of whom the Chief speaks are professionals of irresponsible decisions, in other words, politicians, it is the whole social and political system that must be reevaluated. Industries cannot be held responsible so much, as their charters promise only to make their owners and shareholders rich. It is the governments and those who work there, the elected representatives, who are in charge of preserving and enhancing collective happiness and well being. They are responsible, but are they really accountable? In other parts of the world, a good many of these who took some of the criminal decisions related to past environmental pollution cases are now in other occupations, untouchable by law, protected against just anger or vengeance.

In fact we very rarely have to deal with hardened criminals, malicious in their decision. Most of the time our politicians are only *ignorants* running scared, ducking behind intellectual and reasonable rationalization. It is reasonable according to politicians and industrial leaders to want a strong economy, a prosperous industry and a positive balance of payments. Too bad if to accomplish this it becomes necessary to kill children, poison adults and destroy the environment forever.

How often in our reporting efforts, political, industrial and scientific authorities have advised us to be reasonable, they evidently meant for us to mitigate our criticisms according to the imperatives already mentioned. How many times have we been advised not to show excessive emotion. But what other course do we have when confronted with useless suffering, destruction and death?

One path only, only one course of action remains possible: avoid a discussion based on fabricated inhuman values, and let our instinct cry out. Reason often becomes an excuse to justify incompetence and cupidity, instinct and collective

---

*The "crève-coeur" is a French expression that has no exact English translation. Literally it means "kill-heart". Here is it used in the sense of "heart-breaking."

anger on the other hand express only compassion and thirst for justice and joy.

It is imperative that our elected representatives are made truly responsible and accountable, and that they no longer are permitted to be merely the servants of vested interests. The full employment of a few thousand people does not justify the death or infirmity of a few thousand others.

And may we stop in the name of the gross national product to wipe with money the tears of despair of those sacrificed to the Golden Calf.

Philippe Cousteau
Monaco
March 1977

Philippe Cousteau is vice president in charge of the audio-visual department of the Cousteau Society. As executive producer of one of the society's film series, Oasis in Space, *he was aroused by the story of Grassy Narrows and featured it in "What Price Progress", a segment of the series. The authors and publisher are grateful to him for writing the Foreword to* Grassy Narrows.

Preface

The Ojibway people of Grassy Narrows live in northwestern Ontario on the banks of a river that will be polluted for up to one hundred years. Grandchildren, perhaps even great-grandchildren, of those alive today will have spent their lives before fish from the English River are safe to eat. There is mercury in the English, Wabigoon and Winnipeg river system, and there is nothing anyone can do to remove it; there is no way to hasten the recovery of the waters or to eliminate the poison from the fish.

The consequences of the pollution have been severe for the people of Grassy Narrows, and their neighbours at the Whitedog reserve, fifty miles downstream. Their health has been jeopardized and their economy shattered. Their community reels with social strife. Their plight in the early days of the mercury crisis was largely ignored, drawing little sympathy from the white population in southern Ontario and, consequently, almost no political action. For years they have been paying the price of our environmental neglect.

Perhaps it is because technological man has become hardened, has deluded himself into believing that he has learned to live with industrial pollution in all its forms. But Grassy is not the only area where the ecology has been disrupted and man is threatened. We have chosen to highlight the people of Grassy Narrows, because we know them best and their story is a particularly tragic drama. But the assault of modern technology is the same at hundreds of locations across North America.

Since industrial chemistry began 150 years ago, approximately 2,500,000 different synthetic chemical compounds have been created. About 200,000 of these are currently in commercial production and about three new ones are introduced every day. Many of them, through ignorance or outright negligence, escape the plants in which they are produced or used to work in mysterious, damaging ways in nature.

In Placentia Bay on Newfoundland's southern coast, fish have been found floating on the surface of the sea, red with the phosphorous lost from a chemical plant. Young salmon have difficulty surviving in the Saint John River in New Brunswick, once the third largest salmon run in North America, because of pollution from pulp mills. In Lac Dufault in Quebec, researchers have found high levels of copper, lead, zinc, cadmium, arsenic and mercury from mining operations. Fish in Manitoba's Lake Winnipeg carry mercury, and phosphorous threatens the Qu'Appelle basin near Regina, Saskatchewan with the same fate as Lake Erie. Indians reported as early as 1968 that fish in Pinchi Lake, British Columbia, were dying and in 1975 announced there were no fish left in the lake. Pinchi is about 100 miles north of Prince George, site of a former mercury mine. Zinc has polluted Rose Creek in the Yukon. Indians in Yellowknife have been warned not to melt snow for water because it contains high levels of arsenic. We all suffer for this monstrous abuse, but none have suffered more than the people of Grassy Narrows.

I first developed an interest in mercury pollution while working the environment beat at the London

Free Press where I wrote some of the early stories on the disruption of commercial fishing on Lake St. Clair and in the western basin of Lake Erie. A visit in 1971 to north-western Ontario made a lasting impact on me, shaking my sense of objectivity with the realization that even this wonderful wilderness retreat was polluted – and would remain so for generations. In 1972 I was assigned to cover the Ontario Legislature. From the lofty vantage point of the press gallery at Queen's Park, I listened to the often strident debate over mercury and its effects on the two Indian reserves in the northwest. It was a quiet question, however, which focused my attention on the Indians. A New Democrat wanted to know details about the death of Tom Strong, a forty-two-year-old Ojibway fishing guide who had collapsed while on a rice-harvesting expedition from Grassy Narrows. The cause of Strong's death was officially listed as a heart attack, but the people of Grassy feared he was Ontario's first victim of what the Japanese called "Minamata Disease", mercury poisoning.

The government's response to the question did not satisfy me. Cabinet ministers assured their political combatants across the aisle that everything was being done that could be done to respond positively to the pollution crisis in the northwest. But when I telephoned Grassy Narrows and talked with Bill Fobister, who was at that time serving as the band's administrator, I was told the people continued to eat regular meals of poisoned fish from the contaminated waterways: "We don't know what

danger there is," he said. His comment was a condemnation of both provincial and federal governments. Well over two years had passed since the discovery of the poison. By 1972, the decade-old Japanese experience had been well documented – more than one hundred persons having paid with their lives for eating mercury-contaminated seafood, and thousands more maimed. I knew I had to pursue the story, had to find out what danger there was, not suspecting that the pursuit in the years ahead would take me across the province and halfway around the world.

I returned to London in 1974 as an investigative reporter and, in the early months of 1975, began working on a series of articles on mercury in Ontario, a review of the preceding five years. Photographer Dick Wallace and I teamed up to tell the story for *Free Press* readers. During the long hours, days and weeks spent researching the mercury series, the trips to Grassy and the moving experience of meeting Minamata Disease survivors and their families in Japan, the seed of this book was planted. We knew that our material had to be brought together so that the entire story of Grassy could be told. Our hope is that the personal tragedies and political intrigues documented in these pages may move the reader to a fuller appreciation of the far-reaching consequences of pollution – and a deeper concern for the imminent danger we all face.

G.H.
London, Ontario
February, 1977

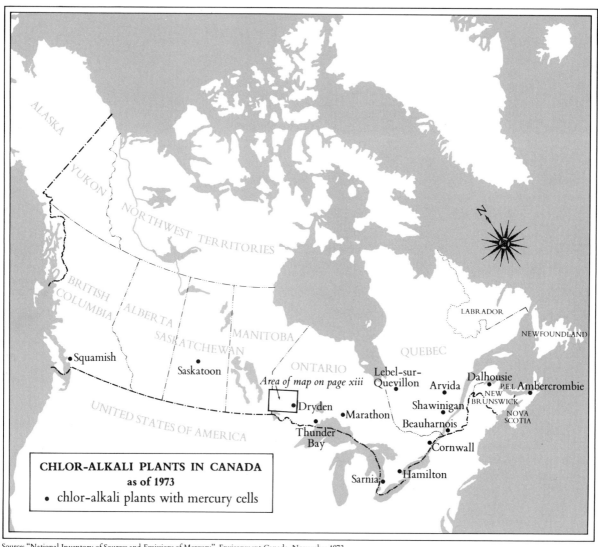

CHLOR-ALKALI PLANTS IN CANADA
as of 1973
• chlor-alkali plants with mercury cells

ALASKA

YUKON

NORTHWEST TERRITORIES

BRITISH COLUMBIA

ALBERTA

SASKATCHEWAN

MANITOBA

ONTARIO

QUEBEC

LABRADOR

NEWFOUNDLAND

• Squamish

• Saskatoon

Area of map on page xiii

• Dryden

• Marathon

Thunder Bay

Lebel-sur-Quevillon

Arvida

Shawinigan

Beauharnois

Cornwall

Dalhousie

P.E.I.

Ambercrombie

NEW BRUNSWICK

NOVA SCOTIA

Sarnia

• Hamilton

UNITED STATES OF AMERICA

Source: "National Inventory of Sources and Emissions of Mercury", Environment Canada, November 1973

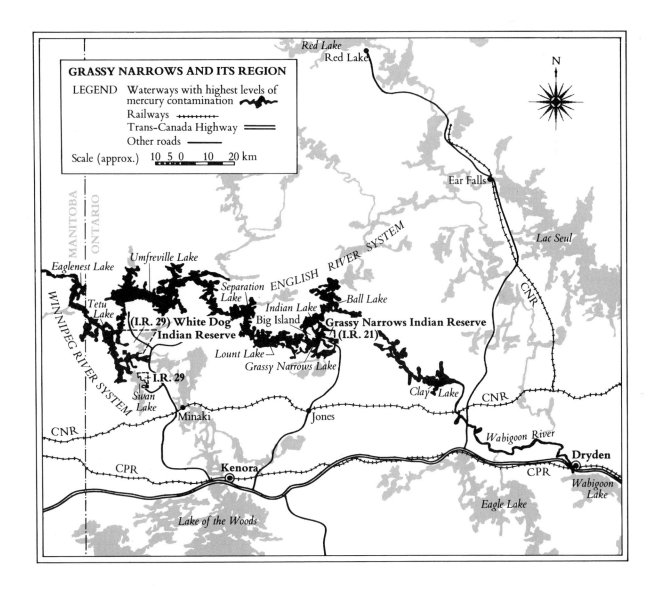

GRASSY NARROWS AND ITS REGION

LEGEND   Waterways with highest levels of
mercury contamination
Railways
Trans-Canada Highway
Other roads

Scale (approx.)   10 5 0   10   20 km

Red Lake
Red Lake

N

Ear Falls

Lac Seul

CNR

MANITOBA
ONTARIO

Eaglenest Lake

Umfreville Lake

Separation
Lake

ENGLISH RIVER SYSTEM

Tetu
Lake

Ball Lake

Indian Lake

**(I.R. 29) White Dog
Indian Reserve**

Big Island

Grassy Narrows Indian Reserve

WINNIPEG RIVER SYSTEM

Lount Lake

(I.R. 21)

Grassy Narrows Lake

I.R. 29

Clay Lake

CNR

Swan
Lake

Minaki

Jones

Wabigoon River

CNR

Dryden

CPR

Kenora

CPR

Wabigoon
Lake

Lake of the Woods

Eagle Lake

Sharon Fobister at her brother's grave.

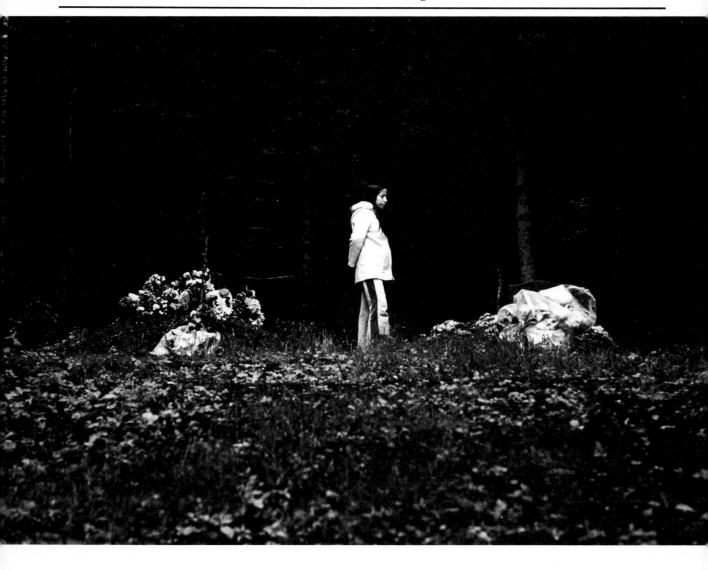

1
Days
of Change

This old blind man, he used to say pretty soon we will have nothing. He said the white people will dirty our waters so bad, our rivers, that we won't be able to drink the water. They will spoil the fish. They will destroy the world and all of us are going to be blind.

—Andy Keewatin,
Grassy Narrows, 1976

Sharon Fobister ran through the darkness to her brother Patrick, who was lying face down on the ground outside House Number Fourteen. She dropped to her knees and searched for signs of life, gently touching his cheek and stroking his sandy hair. In the October chill, he was warm against her fingers, but in the dim light which shone from a curtainless window, he was motionless, and she wailed for her sixteen-year-old "little" brother. Sharon was oblivious to the drunken confusion around her. She stayed by Patrick's side until a cousin, Bill Fobister, mercifully covered the boy's body with a blanket and led her away.

The investigation by the Ontario Provincial Police (OPP) was swift and thorough. A fourteen-year-old boy was arrested, tried and dispatched to reformatory for the shooting death of Patrick Fobister.

The people of Grassy Narrows were troubled, but unsurprised by Patrick's murder. Violence and death had become as much a pattern of life at Grassy as the seasons — changeable but predictable. Patrick's death in October 1974 was preceded months earlier by the killing of an infant whose body was found floating near the shore of Garden Lake, near his home. The mother was charged. In the following few months a thirteen-year-old boy was stabbed to death, a baby was left in a snowbank to die from exposure, a thirty-year-old man bled to death from knife wounds and the body of an old man was found on the rutted gravel road which connected the reserve to the highway to Kenora, fifty miles south. His head had been crushed by a rock.

Each crime was alcohol-related. In a moment of frustration, OPP Corporal Bill Bailey concluded: "We'll never change them. It'll be like this a hundred years from now." Bailey's four-man detachment had been given the job of bringing order back to the wilderness community of nearly five hundred Ojibway. If the objective appeared beyond reach at times, it was not without reason. Family fights, woundings by firearms, knives and clubs provided frequent evidence of the social chaos which had overtaken Grassy.

One distraught ten-year-old girl stole two rifles from her enraged and drunken father, smashed them on a rock and flung the shattered parts into the bush to protect her mother from attack. When the father began flailing the mother with a two-by-four plank, the girl's younger brother slammed a hubcap against his father's head, opening a deep wound. Both parents needed medical treatment.

During such violent outbreaks on the reserve, fearful children often took refuge at a nearby lodge operated by Mennonites. Or, like their parents, they found intoxicants of their own to escape the reality of their existence. They sniffed solvents and gasoline. "That's a real problem," the policeman said. "We don't know what to do about it."

Andy Keewatin, three-term chief of the Ojibway band at Grassy Narrows, tried to explain. "Ever since mercury," he said, "there's been quite a change. You never used to see any murders. There's been a lot of drinking, too. We didn't use to."

The people of Grassy Narrows were already struggling with the social disruption that followed the relocation of their village when they were dealt another staggering blow — mercury from pulp and paper operations upstream was discovered in fish from the English River system in the spring of 1970. Like a sand castle assaulted by waves, the reserve's economy was undermined. Scores of fishing guides lost their jobs when two tourist lodges closed. Commercial fishermen were not allowed to sell their catch. Overnight, Grassy was transformed into a welfare community besieged by enormous social, political and medical problems. In addition, medical examinations and laboratory analyses confirmed that the people of Grassy, and residents of the Whitedog reserve fifty miles further downriver, were carrying potentially dangerous levels of mercury in their bodies.

Grassy Narrows did not stand alone as an Indian community in turmoil. From Moosonee to Red Lake, reserves in Ontario and across Canada were drowning in alcohol. Violence was commonplace. Statistics revealed that Indians in the Kenora district were dying at an astonishing rate of more than one every week, and most of the deaths were tied to alcohol in some way — murder, exposure, suicide, car crashes. But nowhere had circumstances conspired so tragically against the native people as at Grassy.

In the years immediately preceding and following the discovery of mercury in the waterway, Grassy experienced a marked jump in its death rate to almost one in every fifty persons, about three times the national average. Many counted in the annual toll were newborn infants and young babies, leading the people to suspect an attack by mercury on pregnant women on the reserve. Lacking scientific knowledge about the workings of mercury on the human body, the people also suspected it might have something to do with the violent behavior in recent years.

"I think it is a contributing factor," said Dr. Peter Newberry, noting that irritability can be increased as mercury invades the brain and central nervous system. Newberry, a retired physician with the air wing of the Canadian Armed Forces, was sent by the Society of Friends (Quakers) and the National Indian Brotherhood to study the impact of mercury at Grassy. "I'm fairly well convinced that the direct medical effects of mercury play a significant part in the picture. . . . Just looking at the population, you can't say that mercury has done this to the people, because it's such a vague kind of thing. But they have the blood levels which, it has been shown, have these effects in industrial populations."

Newberry had no data to support his conclusion. No research had been done, or has been done, to trace the violent effects of mercury in tandem with alcohol. But the suspicion persisted, despite the prevailing white view that Indians simply "can't hold their liquor."

"They're always drunk," said the wife of one fishing lodge operator in the area. "They've been killing their kids before mercury was ever found. Cats starving to death. Kids with bloated stomachs. So don't blame it on mercury . . . They've always been like that. You have Indians in Toronto; they can't drink. None of them can. So, everything that happens they blame on mercury, which isn't right."

Such attitudes had some basis in the hard reality of northern life. Many native people liked intoxicants and tended to drink to excess. It had been so for centuries. Alcohol became a disruptive influence on Indian life with the arrival of the white man in North America. The machinery of the fur trade, which supported the early stages of colonization of the New World, was lubricated with liquor. Europeans carried it with them into the interior as a valuable commodity for barter. Jesuit missionaries worried about its abuse, as well they might. Indians frequently sold a season of trapping for a secure supply. Many trappers returning from a profitable trip would leave their families destitute by squandering their earnings on liquor. And there was the terrible violence.

The early Jesuits observed: "When these people are intoxicated, they become so furious that they break and smash everything in their houses; they utter horrible yells and shouts, and, like madmen, seek their enemies to stab them. At such times, even their relatives and friends are not safe from their fury, and they bite off one another's noses and ears."

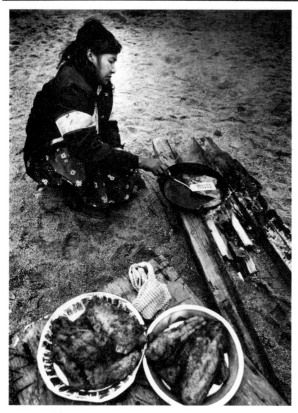

Nora Keewatin, Grassy Narrows.

Why? That question has never been resolved. Some believe Indians see themselves as exceptional persons under the influence of alcohol, allowed to commit violent deeds. Others note that the use of substances which promote dreamlike experiences is more acceptable in the Indian culture.

More often, however, the belief is expressed that Indians tend to drink excessively in response to the heavy pressures placed upon them by the changing nature of their society. Mario Faveri, a community development officer with the Addiction Research Foundation of Ontario, said: "There is no evidence that the Indian is inherently susceptible to intoxication or alcoholism. The alcohol-related problems among native people are the result of historical, social and cultural factors and not due to metabolic or constitutional difference."

Nineteen-year-old Sharon Fobister, however, was living in the present, not the past. She groped for reasons why her people were dying. Her brother Patrick may have been killed by the shot from a rifle wielded by a drunken youngster, but in her mind he was as much a victim of mercury as a bullet.

"There must be something that's causing it," she said. "There are more violent deaths than a few years ago. But I don't know why. I can't say. I don't know how mercury affects people's minds. Mercury must have something to do with it."

Andy Keewatin, the fifty-three-year-old chief of Grassy Narrows, could remember better times, back at the old village along the English River, when alcohol was a minor indulgence which did not

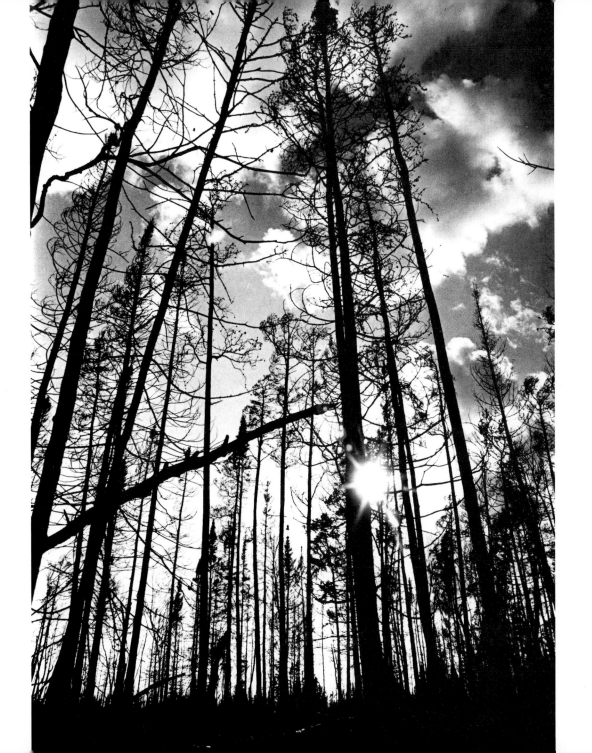

dominate the life of the community. Time was occupied with gaining the basic necessities for survival in the beautiful but harsh environment.

People whose lives began at the old village, as Patrick Fobister's had, once felt blessed. Their eyes opened on an awesome landscape of granite, water and sky. Northwestern Ontario. The English River, a current of narrows and lakes which avoided the Great Lakes on a rambling course towards Hudson Bay, concealed a harvest of walleye, jack fish, lake trout, bass and bottom feeders, and supported a useful crop of waterfowl. Bushes, breaking through stubborn spring snow, soon bowed beneath the weight of succulent berries, and the surrender of the ice to the sun signaled the return of fresh fillets after a season of smoked fish. In the late summer, as reds and golds tipped all but the pines, wild rice waved in the shallows, inviting harvest. Even in the harshest winters, hardy hunters and trappers brought home game and profits from plush animal pelts.

The people enjoyed a wild Eden, abundant in deer, moose, beaver, fish and geese. Energy had to be spent for the harvest. Proper respect for the environment was the only other payment required. Yet respect was commanded by the sheer majesty of the place, an expanse of the world's oldest rock, unveiled by glaciers ten thousand years ago.

The Ojibway were drawn to the region by the abundance of wildlife and the arrival of European fur traders in the 1600s. The Indians drifted with the wildlife populations, delicately sustained by nature's whims and white man's wages. The fur traders were followed into the territory by settlers who squatted on Indian lands. The pernicious invasion had begun. As agents of foreign kingdoms discovered the Ojibway bounty, they sought to buy it with gifts and promises. The promises, some kept, some violated, were not formalized until October 1873, when chiefs and headmen of the Saulteaux and Lac Seul tribes signed what was dispassionately entitled Treaty Number Three by representatives of Her Gracious Majesty Queen Victoria.

The treaty was one of a series negotiated by the government of Canada's first prime minister, John A. Macdonald. His vision of a Confederation from Atlantic to Pacific depended on the construction of a railway through Indian hunting and fishing grounds beyond the Great Lakes and across the prairies. In return for lands to be reserved for farming, fishing and trapping, some farm implements, ammunition and education, the Ojibway surrendered fifty-five thousand square miles —"more or less," in the wording of the treaty. The tract included parts of what are now the provinces of Ontario and Manitoba.

Under the agreement, each of the estimated twenty-five hundred native persons inhabiting the area became a Treaty Indian and was given a twelve-dollar "present" and promised the further sum of five dollars each year for the "extinguishment of all claims." As an inducement to sign the treaty quickly, each of the twenty-four Indian leaders marking his "X" received an annual salary of twenty-five dollars, a flag, commemorative medal, and a "suitable suit of clothing" every three years.

For their part, the chiefs "on their own behalf and on behalf of all other Indians inhabiting the tract within ceded" did "solemnly promise and engage to strictly observe this treaty, and also to conduct and behave themselves as good and loyal subjects of Her Majesty the Queen."

The "rights" to hunting and fishing secured by the ancestors of Patrick Fobister were conditional on the whims and behavior of the government in Ottawa, secure only so long as the land was not required for more lucrative endeavors such as settlement, mining and forestry.

Treaty Three made no promise that Indians would be protected against the antagonistic acts of white men, but did warn that they would be punished for any abuse of whites or their property. The Chiefs were told to "aid and assist the officers of Her Majesty in bringing to justice and punishment any Indian offending against the stipulation of this treaty . . ."

The treaty forbade the sale or introduction of intoxicating liquors on the reserves and vowed that laws passed to protect the Indians "from the evil influences of the use of intoxicating liquors, shall be strictly enforced."

Patrick's people retreated to the supposed safety of the 10,244-acre "Indian Reserve Number 21" at Grassy Narrows on the English River, one of sixty-one reserves set aside for the twenty-five Ojibway bands in the Treaty Three area.

The English River had its source in headwaters to the east, gaining strength from scores of lakes and rivers, including the Wabigoon River. Together, they coursed west, forming more lakes en route to the Winnipeg River and Lake Winnipeg, then

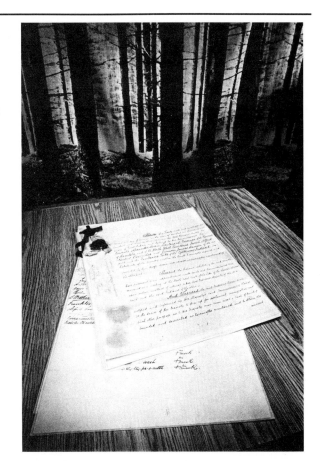

Treaty Three.

following a northerly drift through the land of the Cree, up the Nelson River to the great bay of Hudson.

Grassy Narrows was a serene spot, drawing its name from the quiet, shallow coves, which in summer were carpeted with reeds, lilies and rice shoots. The clean waters served to divide or link the people of Grassy, as they chose. The channels, bays and white-capped open stretches of water offered seclusion to the families who clustered on plateaus, in homesteads hacked from the forest. The waters also provided passage to other clearings in the scattered "village". The people were busy with their own concerns and did not often congregate. But when they did, the occasion was usually happy and conversation was sometimes enhanced by a pot of homebrew made from vegetable or fruit mash.

A favorite meeting place was the council house, built of logs by the people of Grassy on a central rise of land. Another was the Hudson's Bay Company store, on the perimeter of the reserve, a mile or two boating distance. The men talked while the women shopped. The "Bay" was an ever-present influence, granted an awesome charter by the Crown of Great Britain in 1670 to barter with Indians and exploit the resources of the watershed from which it drew its well-known name. A similarly influential presence was the Roman Catholic church, set in a glade, not far from the council house.

Events unfolded naturally here, unhurried. Time was read in seasons on Nature's face. Days began at first light and ended at dusk, the days blending into months and seasons whose passing was marked by the changing patterns of life. "When it was berry picking time," said Andy Keewatin, "we went and picked berries. When it was wild rice time, we went and picked rice. There were no camps, no tourists at that time, so we just moved around."

The airplane brought the future to Grassy Narrows, altering, though not destroying, the seasonal nature of things. Destruction would come later.

In the years following the Second World War, tourism hit the region as flying sportsmen found their way into previously inaccessible lakes. Fishing and hunting lodges sprung up along the Wabigoon and English River chain; the paying guests arrived by pontoon aircraft or logging roads. About two hundred and twenty-five Indians from Grassy and Whitedog took jobs as guides at the seventeen commercial lodges on the chain.

Some men continued to trap and berries were still harvested, but now a more significant sign of spring was Keewatin's departure for Barney's Ball Lake Lodge, located about ten miles up the river, a luxurious camp built by Minnesota-born businessman Barney Lamm in the post-war years to cater to sportsmen who fled offices and factories for controlled excursions into the wilderness. Lamm's lodge was a big business, employing as many as seventy-five persons from Grassy Narrows. Another twenty-five usually worked at the Separation Lake camp, operated by Mr. and Mrs. Colin Myles, a few miles further down the chain.

The airplane also enabled the Indians to tap other southern markets. A commercial fishing industry was started, which increased both the number and diversity of jobs available to the native people. The fishing ventures gave Grassy a thriving economy, by northern standards at least. Pockets were filled with a steady income, and often emptied in the Hudson's Bay store. It was an easy way to earn money. The men had an intimate knowledge of the waters. They knew where the lunkers abounded in the recesses of the river.

But the course of their lives had been changed. They had abandoned their subsistence lifestyle for one tied to wages, and they had based it almost totally on fish. Fewer men found it necessary to trap, or hunt, or gather wild rice. Fewer gardens were planted as increasingly produce was bought from the Bay. Still, there were those who clung to traditional practices. Families, like that of Tom Strong, would paddle canoes into the shallows each August, deftly showering the craft with rice, destined for sale to city gourmet shops and exclusive restaurants. A dozen or so men resisted the temptation to hang up their snowshoes. Each winter, as the snow deepened, men like Joe Loon would resolutely strap on the webbing and stride off to tend thirty or forty miles of trap lines. Days were spent skinning animals and resetting traps. Nights were spent in the snowy silence, warmed by a fire that bounced waves of heat off a nearby bluff.

Whether it was acknowledged or just unconsciously accepted, the people of Grassy Narrows had climbed upon a precarious perch, balanced somewhere between progress and the past. Although they remained largely isolated from the society beyond the boundaries of the reserve, they were becoming increasingly dependent on it for survival.

December 11, 1957. A midwife delivered Patrick Fobister into the uncertain and changing world of Grassy Narrows, the last of six Fobister children. His short life would be as turbulent as his people's. When he was four years old, his parents separated, and for the next ten years he would be raised as a transient between white and native cultures, moving with his brothers, sisters and mother off the reserve. His oldest brother, Andrew, found work along the mainline of the Canadian National Railways, and supported the family. They lived in cabins and tents, in communities with names like McIntosh and Jones.

Back at Grassy, further change was overtaking Patrick's people, signaling the beginning of a foreign way of life, but necessary, they were told. In the early part of the 1960s, the federal government approached the band council to suggest that the people move from the old village to a new location, within the reserve boundaries but four or five miles away. Ottawa's details of the proposal are sketchy, but a logging road was being extended northward and the Hudson's Bay Company wanted to relocate. The government saw it as an appropriate time to propose a wholesale move to the community.

Relocation would enable the government to fulfill some of the promises unfulfilled since the signing of Treaty Three, namely the provision of schooling for the children of the reserve. Other amenities would also be provided, the people of Grassy were told — electricity, running water. The prospect of a school had particular appeal to them.

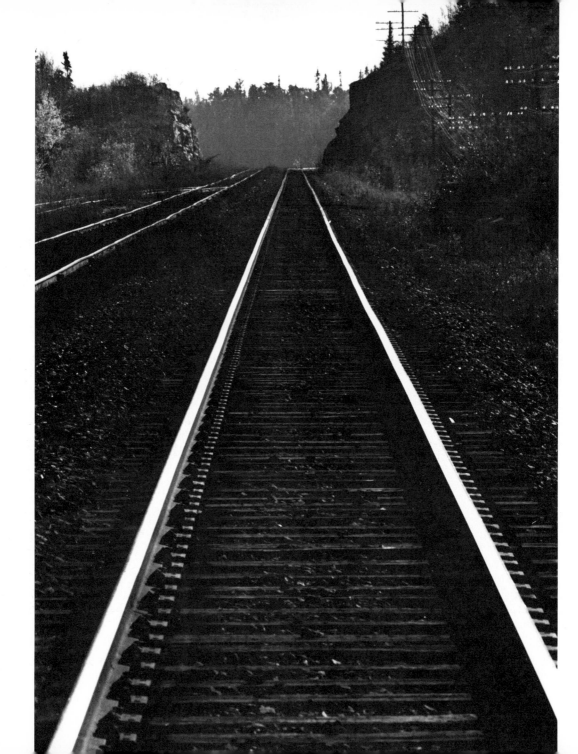

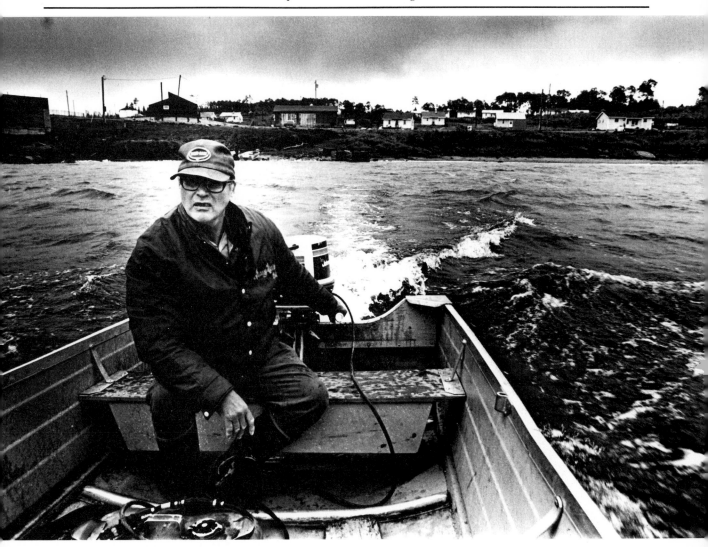

Canadian National mainline in northern Ontario (left).
Andy Keewatin at the new village.

Dennis Clark, Grassy Narrows school principal.

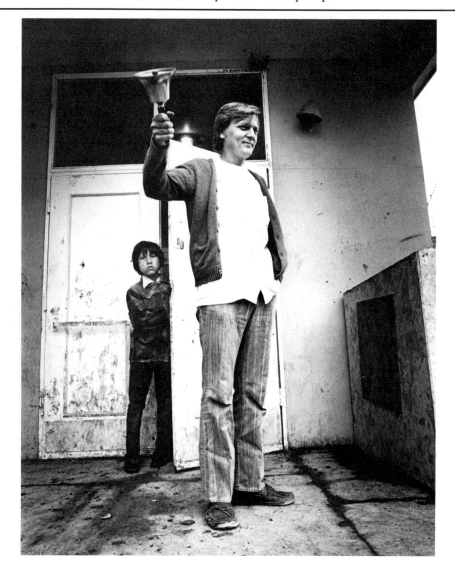

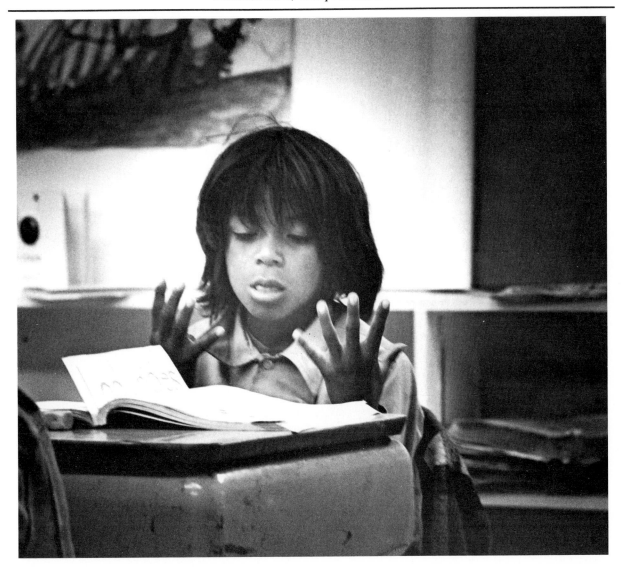

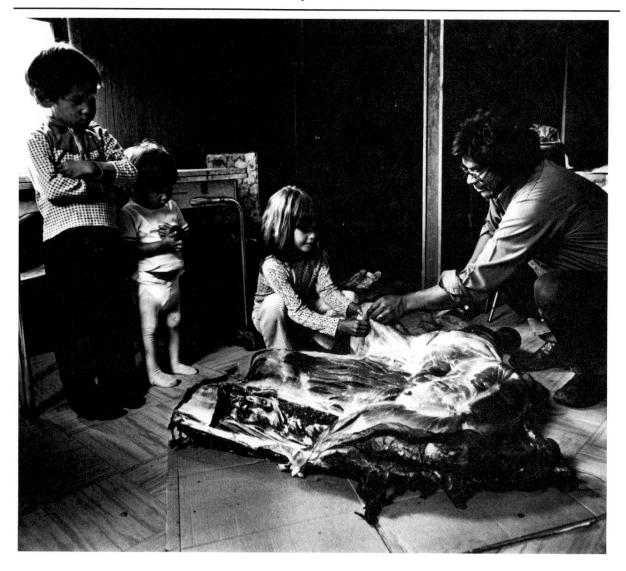

If we want our kids educated, we have to lose something.
Andy Keewatin

If their children were to cope with their changing world, education was vital. Formal education in any real sense was fifty miles away in Kenora, the logging and tourist center along Lake of the Woods. Until now, parents who insisted upon having their children schooled had to move off the reserve or send their youngsters away. Most remained at home, uneducated.

Besides, there were disadvantages to sending children to Kenora. A growing community of about ten thousand persons which depended heavily on tourism and pulp and paper for its economic well-being, Kenora had lost none of its flavor as a frontier town. There was often friction as Indians from nearby reserves came to town to shop, have fun, drink in the bars. Some white merchants openly discriminated against the natives. In 1965, native people staged a march on the town to protest their second-class treatment.

Life would be better at Grassy at a new location, the government told the people. The logging road was being extended from the railway junction at Jones, twenty miles south, and could easily be directed into the reserve, for the first time providing direct road access to the outside world. The people were told the government would build a school and finance new homes, like the ones in town. No longer would the people of Grassy Narrows have to live in log cabins in the bush. The good life was waiting, just four or five miles away.

The people resisted relocation. They feared losing their traditional way of life and were disturbed by the design of the new village, with its prefabricated buildings laid out in symmetrical patterns of congestion. They debated the advantages and disadvantages. The people were proud of the old village. It had been built by them. They had constructed the council house and the church and the cabins among the trees. There was space, a sense of freedom and privacy. Their ancestors were buried there. The new village, however, would have electric power, radios and television sets, running water. The Bay store would be a walk away. And there would be a school.

The government did not force relocation on the people, but the promises were very attractive. In 1963, when Andy Keewatin packed up his family and moved, debate was at an end. "If we want our kids educated," Keewatin reasoned, "we have to lose something." One by one, the people followed. The new village was built in stages, and it took years to construct houses for everyone.

Patrick Fobister was among the first youngsters to attend the new school. His family returned to Grassy in 1965 and, at the age of eight, he attended school for the first time with his own people. He may have felt more at home, but the lessons at school were still confusing, structured as they were on white values.

"They were taught in English, when most of the kids speak Ojibway at home," Grassy Narrows school principal Dennis Clark explained. "The kids were set back two years automatically. Language is the framework of their concepts, and there are concepts in Ojibway for which there are no words in English. And there are concepts in English that were foreign concepts to these kids.

"The Dick and Jane readers are gone. Now, it's Bill and Jill and Ken, but Bill and Jill and Ken live in the city and they have black friends and Chinese friends."

Patrick's stay at Grassy was brief. His mother remarried and, in 1966, the Fobisters moved to Dryden, eighty miles from the reserve on the Wabigoon River, a typical northern logging town whose prosperity was tied to the fortunes of the Dryden Pulp and Paper Company and its sister chemical plant. Town residents had to put up with the company's outfall into the Wabigoon — a frothing, foul-smelling effluent that killed off fish for miles below the plant. No one was aware that wastes from the chemical plant were building up in the fish far downstream at Grassy Narrows.

Patrick tolerated school in Dryden, but turned inward, confused by the contradictions around him. "The Indian who is subjected to white education," social scientist Robert Havighurst once wrote, "becomes a man of two cultures. Sometimes the Indian culture predominates and sometimes the white culture wins. Generally, the individual makes his own combination of the two by adopting such white 'ways' as are useful and pleasant to him, including farming and homemaking skills, artisan skills and often a form of Christianity."

Patrick found expression in painting and drawing. At an early age, his scrawls assumed familiar shapes of lakes and shores, trees, boats, sunrises, trains disturbing the northern wilderness. His drawing showed enough promise that by the time he had reached his thirteenth birthday at Dryden, a professional artist was providing him with materials and encouragement to paint pictures for profit. He sold one or two, but gave up the "business" when his family moved once again, back to Grassy, for the final time.

Patrick, now a strapping boy of fourteen returned to find the reserve, and the people, torn by strife. Mercury had been discovered two years earlier in fish from the English River and dangerously high levels of the contaminant had been detected among some fishing guides. Two of the major fishing camps were closed and commercial fishing had been banned. Grassy's fledgling economy was destroyed. The federal government funded make-work projects, but unemployment approached 80 per cent. The community depended heavily on welfare. Many used the payments to buy booze, creating severe social tensions which frequently flared into violence.

In the years since relocation of the village, the death rate had been climbing, particularly among infants. Four newborn babies died in 1966, six in 1967, two in 1968, three in 1969, all of unexplained causes. In 1970, the year in which the economy was shattered by the loss of the fishing trade, eight deaths were recorded on the reserve. The total included two gunshot deaths and two by exposure. In 1971 there were ten deaths, including two in a fire and one by drowning.

The medical impact of mercury pollution on Grassy Narrows would become a matter of rigorous political and public debate for years, but the social

> **The social problems that exist on these reserves,**
> **although not directly attributable to mercury,**
> **have been intensified....** *Judd Buchanan*

impact was unmistakable and devastating. Officials of the Addiction Research Foundation (ARF) of Ontario witnessed a significant jump in the number of people from Grassy being arrested as common drunks on the streets of Kenora. Numbers also increased at the waystation for troubled natives that had been opened by ARF following the 1965 march, at the request of the Indian people. The townspeople called the center the "Indian Tank." The Children's Aid Society was summoned to care for more youngsters from Grassy, the products of broken homes, and the Ontario government moved to establish a police detachment near the reserve.

In just a few years, the people of Grassy Narrows had been transformed into convenient stereotypes — drunken Indians. The view was seldom expressed publicly, but it was commonly held that the Indians' problem was not mercury but booze. A few people knew better.

Indian Affairs Minister Judd Buchanan, the federal cabinet minister charged with the responsibility of safeguarding the rights of Canada's native peoples, blamed pollution of the waterway for severely disrupting the "cycle of life" at both Grassy and the neighboring Whitedog reserve.

"The social problems that exist on these reserves, although not directly attributable to mercury, have been intensified by the elimination of many jobs related to the tourist industry," he said. "Feelings of victimization and helplessness, while not unique to these reserves, have also been heightened by the fact that a serious health threat exists."

One anthropologist has referred to Indian drinking as the longest protest demonstration in the world, a conscious reaction to the way in which white society has overrun their traditional culture. Others suggest that failure by whites to understand the causes of native alcoholism has perpetuated the drinking problem. Prevailing wisdom, however, explains native drinking as a response to severe stress from external pressure. In this sense, Grassy Narrows was a classic case. Whatever explanation one chooses, it is essential that it not be forgotten that these are people, like all of us, struggling with life.

Patrick, like many teenagers today, refused to remain in school. He managed to land a job on a building project at the village. He became a construction worker, and helped clear the bush for the long-promised power line being strung up from the south.

"He could have continued school," said Sharon Fobister, "but he was very sensitive. When he came back here he was bigger than all the kids who were going to school. He was almost a man, and all the kids were small. Kids his size were all working, so he started working." He devoted his leisure time to his paintings, and a car, bought for him by his doting mother. "I guess you would say he was spoiled," said Sharon. "He didn't go around saying 'Look what my mom bought for me,' but he did get mostly what he wanted. My mom bought him a second-hand car and he had these expensive cameras, record player and a stack of records; rock, the kind you can't even understand."

Patrick invested hours on the car, an old clunker. He tore it apart and restored it to running

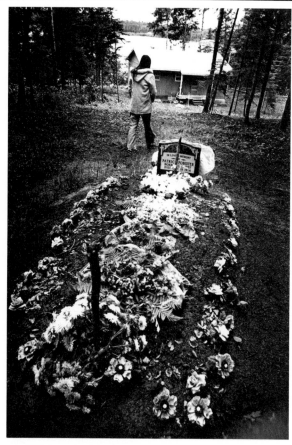

The grave of Patrick Fobister.

order. He used it to run a taxi service to the Bay, picking up pin money. At night, he would withdraw to his bedroom where he would sketch to the sound of his rock records, and his family would tell him to turn the sound down.

Occasionally, he would allow his sister into his inner sanctum. Though Sharon was three years his senior, married with a child of her own, they were much alike, secretive of their thoughts. They would talk about what they saw, what might be, warm images of better times.

"I was the only one he would really talk to," said Sharon. "We were very close...

"The night he was shot, we attended a movie. It started around nine o'clock in the rec' hall. My husband had left on a fishing trip and my little brother came to get me to go to the movie.

"My mother made a mistake and drank that day. Patrick didn't like it when our parents drank. He was very close to his mom and whenever she did bad, he felt bad. They had all been drinking that day and he came to me. He said she went to town that morning and was supposed to come back to the band office... We picked up mom and drove her home. Later, we went to the movie together."

Following the movie, "I told him he had better go straight home. He said okay. I went to bed before the late show was over... Then somebody was pounding on the door. He said 'Patrick has been shot. I think Patrick is dead.' I put on my shoes and started running.

"I saw my little brother lying there, a few steps from the front of the house. He wasn't moving and

I started losing my mind. I knelt down beside him. He seemed so still. I was kinda scared to touch him, because I didn't want to have to feel him. I touched his face, and he didn't seem that cold right then. I was crying and I was scared, because I was alone. Everyone else just took off. I just stayed there.

"My brother Steve showed up. He asked if Patrick was dead. No one actually wanted to find out if he was dead. But as I was sitting there for nearly an hour I knew he was dead because he wasn't breathing . . .

"One of the biggest funerals we have had was my little brother's funeral," said Sharon. "We had a church service. It was just packed. Some people were outside. There must have been twenty cars and trucks. Generally, when you call a meeting here, you don't see that many people. He was well loved by the people."

Patrick's mother picked a grave site on the hill overlooking her home. Men cleared the area, creating a pine-shaded shrine within view of her window. She adorned the grave with plastic flowers that would maintain their color through Grassy's changing seasons. She had a granite headstone prepared to mark his grave.

IN LOVING MEMORY
OF
PATRICK FOBISTER
BORN DEC. 11, 1957
DIED OCT. 16, 1974

"She says her baby will always be there, close," said Sharon. "He was the baby, the favorite. He was the closest to everybody. Before his death, my mother wanted to move off the reserve. But since he died, there's no way you could pull her off this reserve. That is where he is lying, and that is where she will remain."

Sharon said her mother did not want Patrick buried in the new cemetery, or over at the old village.

"Mom wanted him here so she could be near him, to take care of him. The others, over there, are forgotten."

2
Mercury
and
Its Victims

The first evidence of a mercury crisis in Canada was discovered a thousand miles away from Grassy Narrows, far to the southeast, in the Lake St. Clair region of the Great Lakes chain.

March 23, 1970, an appropriately chilling day. The wind whipped out of the west under ashen skies in a last frigid gasp of winter, and it cut through the heavy jackets of the St. Clair fishermen. But it was at their backs and their cumbersome "pound net" boats slammed forward against the waves and melting ice floes. Though the weather was raw, the men were exuberant. The season had opened well. The two boats rode low in the water, straining beneath a full cargo of pickerel and perch, most of it bound for United States markets. Dime Jubenville figured the catch for the day should bring in about $3,000.

Scooter, the Labrador retriever, sat high in the bow of the lead boat, barking at the waves as Dime joked with his two nephews above the roar of the powerful outboards. The boys would share the day's reward. So would Dime's son, Kent, who piloted the second boat. At thirty-one, Kent was the father of four children. He had been a fisherman since his teens, like his father and grandfather before him. He flashed a satisfied grin at his dad, who was also obviously enjoying himself. Dime was happy with his forty-one years on the lake. He had a good home. A son who shared his love of the business. Grandchildren. And he was his own boss.

The commercial fishing industry on Lake St. Clair supported only about fifty families, but it provided a hard-won satisfaction for those willing to invest hours in a pitching, twenty-eight-foot open aluminum boat, straining with aches from hauling heavy nets from the water. Few had completed much more than high school. The only education needed was an appreciation of the lake.

Lake St. Clair can be calm as puddled oil at times, yet ever ready to churn under a brisk breeze. A relative pond among the mighty Great Lakes, it forms part of the border between the United States and Canada at the western end of southern Ontario. Between Lake St. Clair and Lake Huron, the St. Clair River separates the industrial border towns of Port Huron, Michigan, and Sarnia, Ontario. This region is known by natives as the Chemical Valley, because of the predominance of oil refineries and petrochemical industries. From Lake St. Clair to the south, toward Lake Erie, the Detroit River flows, dividing the towering metropolis of Detroit, Michigan, from the low-profile city of Windsor, Ontario.

In the winter, the flatlands around Lake St. Clair were swept by wind and snow. The season was a time of respite to the farmers and fishermen of European ancestry who populated the shores. But as spring approached, the farmers began to work the land and the air currents bore the smell of fish into the ports and tributaries, as inviting to fishermen as a whiff of partridge to a bird dog.

The Jubenvilles attacked the 1970 season vigorously, as usual, gambling that the remaining ice chunks would not damage their equipment. After the nets were cast and lifted full of fish, the men rushed back to Dime's harborfront home at Baptiste Creek, where they packed and tagged the day's haul and loaded it onto a truck. There was time to spare before shipping the catch to the processor and they headed for the Lighthouse Hotel at the mouth of the Thames River for a few beers and plates of fried fish. At that moment, they had never heard of Norvald Fimreite and had no way of knowing that his research was about to change their lives.

In 1970, Fimreite was a graduate student at the University of Western Ontario in London, fewer than one hundred miles from Lake St. Clair. A doctoral candidate in environmental science, he had come to Canada from Norway in 1967. His special area of study was mercury contamination, and his pioneering research would soon turn the quiet, bespectacled thirty-four-year-old scholar into something of a scientific celebrity — an environmental supersleuth.

Few knew, and few cared, about mercury in those days. The public had little appreciation of the liquid metal beyond its use in thermometers. Some had a vague idea that it could be harmful, recognizing the Mad Hatter in Alice in Wonderland as a fairytale parody of nineteenth-century hat makers, demented by mercury while working with felt. The more astute identified mercury as quicksilver, the only metal occurring as a liquid at normal surface temperatures on earth, a curious silvery substance that beaded and shimmered and smeared. Mercury is heavy, thirteen-and-a-half times the weight of water.

But outside the laboratories and factories of commerce, the public was largely unaware of its vital, and often dangerous, presence. It was everywhere. Readily converted to a gas, it entered the atmosphere from hot fissures in the earth's crust. It fell to the ground with rain and snow, and leached from rocky deposits swept by groundwater. Man had learned to live with mercury in its natural cycle. It seldom accumulated beyond trace amounts. But that would change as modern technology hit the western world and chemists discovered useful compounds which required mercury as a component.

In the twentieth century chemical engineers began using mercury in the production of a broad range of goods and it soon had as many as three thousand industrial applications. It found its way into such diverse products as electrical parts, contraceptive jelly, water-based paints, agricultural fungicides, medicines, even cosmetics. It was used to make photographic film and plastics, and in chloralkali plants mercury cells served to break down brine in the production of chlorine and caustic soda, which was used extensively by the pulp and paper industry to bleach fine papers. In addition, large amounts of mercury enter the atmosphere through industrial smokestacks when fossil fuels are burned. The smelting of ores to obtain other metals often releases mercury in the process.

Fimreite came by his interest in mercury naturally. Scandinavia had been hit by mercury pollution as early as 1950, when bird watchers noticed a declining bird population. In 1965, Swedish scientist Gunnel Westöö pinpointed the cause as methyl mercury, widely used as a treatment to protect farm seed from rot. The seed was being consumed in great quantities by wildfowl. Following Westöö's discovery, the Swedish government severely restricted the use of mercury in agriculture.

Fimreite, meanwhile, was monitoring similar research in Norway as secretary with the Norwegian Toxicological Committee on Pesticides. He held the position for three years and recorded the results of a study into the effects of mercury-treated seed on wildlife. The committee learned that mercury in its methylated state attacked the vital organs and reproduction systems of birds. Eggs were laid with shells so thin they would break before hatching. Scientists in both Scandinavian countries also observed a buildup of mercury in fish downstream from some chemical plants and pulp and paper mills, a warning which raised the frightening spectre of Minamata Disease.

Minamata would forever be identified with mercury poisoning. A city of more than fifty thousand persons on Japan's southernmost island of Kyushu, on a bay of the beautiful Shiranui Sea, Minamata was the scene of an ecological disaster in the 1950s and 1960s. Methyl mercury discharged since 1932 by the city's major industry, the petrochemical giant Chisso Corporation, killed at least ninety persons and left thousands more with irreversible injuries — crippled limbs, brain damage, blindness, paralysis, internal disorders, loss of motor functions. The disease inflicted itself most heavily upon poor fishing families in the city and villages along the coast whose diets depended almost totally on seafood. Thousands of people left Minamata and the population fell to about 36,000.

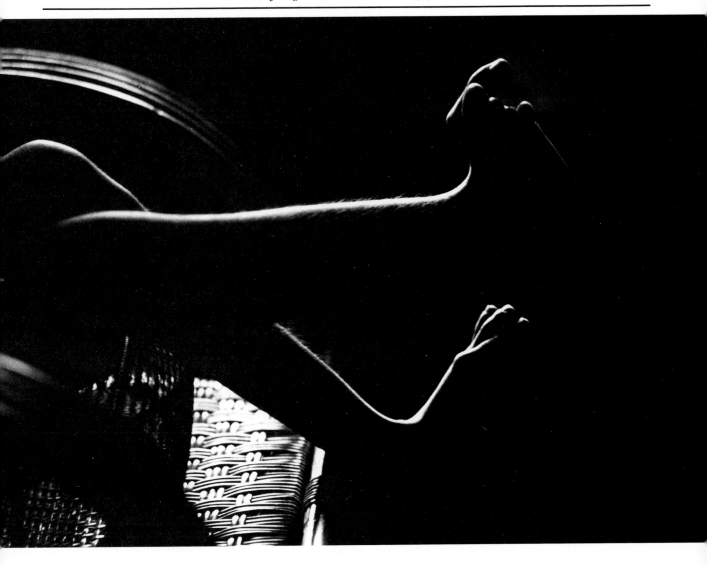

A victim of congenital Minamata Disease, Japan, 1975.

I look on mercury as far more serious than DDT.
Norvald Fimreite

Fimreite feared Canada faced a similar mercury hazard due to its widespread use of the element, particularly in the chlor-alkali industry. He was not alone. Dr. Robert Jervis, a chemist at the University of Toronto, had developed a method of detecting small amounts of metal in food and had visited Sweden and Japan to gather first-hand information on mercury poisoning. In 1966, he was awarded a federal government grant to study the potential emergence of the problem in Canada. Game and health officials were prompted by Jervis' early interest to keep a close eye on Swedish research.

Fimreite, meanwhile, believed hard evidence of mercury contamination could already be found in the Canadian environment. Surrounded by books, stuffed animals and fish tanks in his office at Western, he told a reporter for the London *Free Press* that he believed the threat from mercury was "far more serious than DDT" in "some parts of Canada." His words were a warning, carefully chosen, delivered softly, in a manner that tended to belie their severe ramifications.

The lessons of Minamata had been terrible.

Signs of the poison first appeared in 1950, when fish began to float to the surface of Minamata Bay. They swam erratically and thrashed about before dying. Two years later, people in Minamata and the neighboring villages reported that the strange affliction had attacked their cats. The cats, according to early reports, were committing "suicide." They were taking fits, staggering, squealing, slobbering and spinning recklessly about. Some threw themselves into the sea. Others crashed against walls in a frenzy

before dropping dead. The people, for want of a better name, called it the "cats' dancing disease." Later, it would be known around the world as "Minamata Disease."

In April 1956, a five-year-old girl was taken to the children's ward of the Chisso company hospital. Like the cats, she was suffering from a severe nervous disorder. She could not walk without staggering. She slurred her words. She was often delirious. A month later, a younger sister and four members of a neighboring family were stricken, and Dr. Hajime Hosokawa, head of the Chisso hospital, reported that "an unclarified disease of the central nervous system has broken out."

By mid-summer so many cases had been reported that Dr. Hosokawa and the public health authorities became convinced that they were dealing with a contagious disease. Theories were as numerous as victims. Investigators discovered people who had been ill with the disease since 1953, mistakenly diagnosed as suffering from a variety of maladies such as encephalitis, syphilis, alcoholism, and even some bizarre genetic malfunction.

In August of 1956, the Kumamoto University Medical School organized a research group to track down the precise cause of the disease. They attacked the problem as they would an epidemic, noting the location of the homes of all victims, similarities in their daily movements, medical histories and diets. By October, they had reached the conclusion the so-called disease was not at all infectious; that it was, in fact, a case of mass poisoning, probably traceable to a heavy metal concentrated in the flesh of fish and shellfish in Minamata Bay.

Chisso was a prime suspect. The company every working day poured tons of effluent into the bay, but company officials refused to answer embarrassing questions posed by the scientists and denied them access to the plant. Some scientists entered the plant area without permission to lift samples, but gave them up to company officials for fear of being prosecuted. By action and word, the company denied responsibility and continued to dump its effluent into the bay. Local politicians gave the company their tacit approval — Chisso, after all, was Minamata's major industry, provider of about half of the city's income in salaries and taxes.

It was not until 1962, six full years after the first recorded case of the disease, that scientists were able to positively identify mercury from the Chisso plant as the cause of the outbreak. Through autopsies performed on victims of Minamata Disease and experiments conducted on cats, the scientists from Kumamoto University were able to observe the effects of the poison on vital organs — scientific proof of the consequences of heedlessly tampering with nature. Accompanied by research results in Sweden and the United States, their investigations gradually revealed the deadly course followed by the mercury from the chemical plant to the diets of the people of Minamata.

They discovered that mercury used by Chisso in the production of acetaldehyde and vinyl chloride, substances used in the manufacture of plastics, escaped the production process and became part of waste sludge inside the plant. Bacteria in the sludge transformed the mercury from an inorganic to organic state — into highly toxic methyl mercury, which was dumped with the sludge as effluent into Minamata Bay.

Later, it would be learned the transformation also occurred in nature. Mercury lost directly to waterways in its elemental form would drop to the bottom of rivers and lakes, where bacteria in the mud would methylate it and link the poison to the food chain. The mercury was then absorbed by microscopic underwater life such as plankton or algae, which served as food for insect larvae. The insects were consumed by fish. The mercury was persistent, long lasting and accumulated in its host. It increased in concentration and toxicity as small fish were eaten by larger fish and large fish were eaten by man.

Fish and shellfish from Minamata Bay became highly toxic, with mercury levels commonly running between twenty and thirty parts per million of flesh. The highest level revealed by a living shellfish was forty parts per million. Mud near drainage channels of Chisso was clearly the source of the contamination. Tons of mercury lay in the sediment, feeding a natural mechanism which was pumping poison directly into the diets of thousands of persons up and down the coast. One core sample below the Chisso outfall contained an astonishing mercury level of 2,010 parts per million.

Scientists have not agreed upon what constitutes a lethal dose of mercury. Damage varies with the body weight of individuals consuming the poison and the regularity of intake. However, methyl mer-

**In some cases,
the victims experienced a progressive development of the disease.
In others, the poison appeared to strike almost overnight,
turning healthy fishermen one day into screaming invalids the next.**

cury was found to be so extremely toxic that the U.S. Food and Drug Administration and the World Health Organization decreed that no food should be consumed by humans which contains more than a half part of mercury per million parts of food (.5 ppm), a level accepted as a maximum by federal health authorities in Canada.

In 1967, the World Health Organization stated: "Modern studies of the distribution of mercury in human foods and beverages and in human tissues in different environments and at different ages are urgently required. Until the results of such studies are available, it is not possible to set meaningful maximum permissible limits to dietary intakes of this element. Every effort should therefore be made to control and reduce this form of contamination of the environment and consequently of food."

Over the years of the Minamata "epidemic" the scientists of Kumamoto University documented on film and in text how the consumption of contaminated fish from the bay had affected people. The mercury entered the bloodstream during digestion and was carried to the body's extremities, accumulating along the way in vital organs, particularly the brain, liver and kidneys. The initial effect was much like that from alcohol: minor disruption and damage to nerves and tissues. But after a significant accumulation, the mercury ravaged cells and traumatized organs like a cancer.

Early signs were troublesome, if not worrisome — an almost imperceptible tingling around the lips, on fingertips and toes. But as the poison continued to build and erode brain cells and nerve ends, victims lost their peripheral vision and experienced

tunnel vision. Their body movements became uncoordinated, they staggered. Those who died also experienced blindness, delirium and coma. In some cases, the victims experienced a progressive development of the disease. In others, the poison appeared to strike almost overnight, turning healthy fishermen one day into screaming invalids the next.

The insidious poison worked its terror even among the newborn, penetrating the placental screen of pregnant women to invade the womb and attack the fetus. Minamata recorded forty cases of congenital Minamata Disease, that is children born with gross deformation or severe mental retardation, similar to cerebral palsy. Uncounted children were stillborn. Researchers suspected that even healthy infants could be poisoned as they fed at their mother's breast and ingested crippling levels of mercury.

Yet, despite the mounting evidence, Chisso used its economic and political influence to deflect criticism, and the company continued to dump its untreated, deadly effluent into the waters until 1968. Countless tons of mercury were dumped and scores were killed and maimed before a stop was put to it.

A further sacrifice to industrial ignorance, a second outbreak of Minamata Disease, occurred in 1965 at Niigata, a city north of Tokyo where the Showa Denko Company was discharging vast amounts of mercury. At least twenty-five people died and hundreds more were seriously injured, raising the death toll from mercury poisoning in Japan to at least one hundred and fifteen. Dr. Masazumi Harada, a mercury poisoning diagnostician from Kumamoto University, said more had probably died whose passing had been attributed to other causes. The number lost to Minamata Disease more accurately exceeds two hundred, he said, with injuries totalling, perhaps, ten thousand. The precise toll will never be known.

But the experiences of Minamata and Niigata, and the increasing evidence of mercury pollution elsewhere, appeared of little concern to North Americans. When Norvald Fimreite first arrived in Canada in 1967 he was amazed by the apathy and ignorance displayed by the scientific community regarding the element's threat to the environment. Quite simply, mercury was not viewed as a problem in Canada. Material from Kumamoto University sat in some science libraries, untranslated. At the age of thirty, a doctoral student in a foreign land, Fimreite was doing pioneer research in a field largely ignored by scientists from any of Canada's ten provinces.

Fimreite enrolled at the University of Western Ontario in the fall of 1967, and with supervising professor William Holsworth approached the Canadian Wildlife Service to discuss possible financial and technical support. J. A. Keith, head of the service's pesticide section, suggested research was needed to determine the extent of mercury contamination in Canada and in the spring of 1968 the student ecologist was given a contract which would ultimately provide about $40,000.

In the early stages of his program, Fimreite concluded that the major sources of mercury pollution in Canada were seed dressings containing mercury, pulp and paper mills using mercury slimicides, and chlor-alkali plants with mercury cells. He reported to the wildlife service that although there were only ten chlor-alkali plants operating in Canada, they could be releasing as much as two hundred thousand pounds of mercury every year.

Fimreite based his estimate on a survey conducted among companies that were known users of mercury. He asked them to provide information on annual mercury purchases and estimated losses. Most co-operated with the survey. At least one did not. In December 1968, Fimreite wanted Dow Chemical of Canada at Sarnia on the St. Clair River to provide information on its discharge of mercury. The letter was written by Dr. John George, who had taken over as supervising professor after Dr. Holsworth went to Africa on a field trip. In a letter dated December 18, 1968, J. M. Hacking, Dow's vice-president of public relations, replied: "Your letter regarding the use of mercury in the manufacture of chlorine and its subsequent effect on wildlife has come to my attention. I regret we can be of very little assistance to you on the subject. While both our Sarnia and Fort William plants use the mercury cell process, no effluent is discharged to the surface water."

Hacking's memory was, at best, faulty. Dow's haphazard use of mercury had been on the public record for years. It was raised in debate in the Ontario Legislature as early as 1964, but the issue died without any serious investigation being made into allegations that men were suffering from mercury poisoning and the element was commonly washed down the sewers.

Donald MacDonald, then leader of the pro-labor New Democratic party (NDP), complained in the provincial legislature that men were not

Chisso Corporation plant, Minamata Bay, 1975.

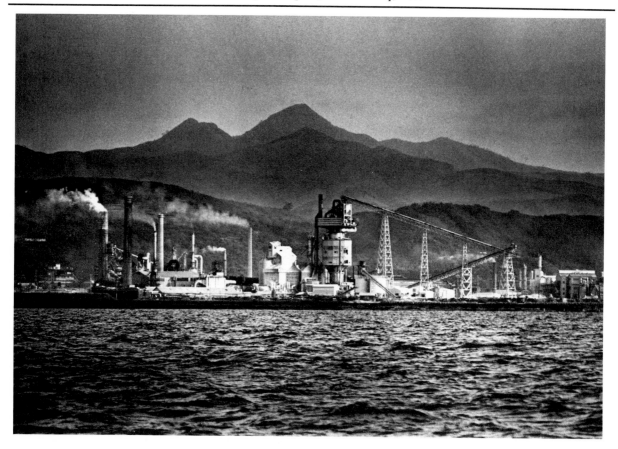

Tsuginori Hamamoto, a Minamata victim, Chisso gates, 1975.

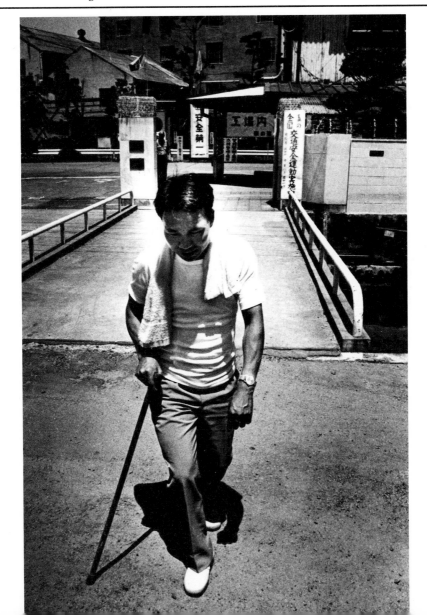

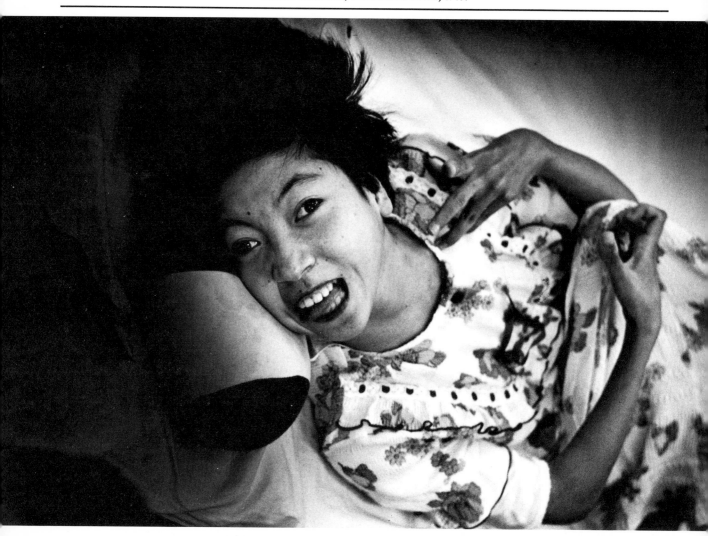

The inspection, according to my information, was a formality and a farce.
Donald MacDonald

qualifying for compensation from the Ontario Workmen's Compensation Board even though Dow's mercury process was damaging their health. Acting on information from a Sarnia labor group, MacDonald claimed the mercury cell installed by Dow in 1949 had only been inspected twice by the Ontario department of health and, on the second occasion at least, the company was given advance notice.

"Officials of the company had prior knowledge of the visit and they proceeded to carry out a thorough and intensified cleaning job," the NDP leader charged. "Grill flooring that had not been inspected for years was removed and all traces of mercury cleaned up. Conditions seen were not normal. No questions were asked, nor any information sought from the working personnel of the department. The inspection, according to my information, was a formality and a farce."

MacDonald said the health of one man in the plant had been so badly affected by mercury that he was transferred to a janitorial job and "his fellow workers . . . are supplementing his income." He quoted a brief from the labor group that charged that "Dow Chemical Company has dragged its feet for twelve years. In the meantime, it has used its workers in the mercury cell plant as guinea pigs."

The brief stated that conditions were so bad inside the plant that in July 1962, "window washers in the mercury cell building found that their brass squeegees became amalgamated and soon disintegrated from the mercury content of the wash water. Analysis of samples of this water revealed a high percentage of mercury. This mercury came from only one source, the air of the building. This is the air the workers on the cell floor have been breathing for years."

MacDonald said mercury readings inside the Dow plant had exceeded allowable levels for years and he criticized the company for refusing to release mercury readings or acknowledge that there was an occupational health problem. He assailed Matthew Dymond, then minister of health, for not acting in the workers' behalf. Dymond took issue with the suggestion that he should be aware of his department's inspection practices at the Dow plant. "I am not advised of every inspection that is carried out by the staff of my department," he told the NDP leader. "This is ridiculous to the extreme to think that such a thing should occur. I would be doing nothing but listening to the reports of these being carried out."

As leader of a party with only a handful of members in the provincial legislature, MacDonald did not expect action from the solidly entrenched Progressive Conservative government. He was right. After much bluster, the matter died with a promise by Dymond that he would study the charges.

Meanwhile, Ralph Knox, the Progressive Conservative (PC) member for the Sarnia riding, felt embarrassed and obliged to act for his wealthy corporate constituent. He wrote to Hacking, the public relations man, and asked advice on how to respond to the NDP leader's allegations in further debate.

"To speak on this," Knox said in a letter later intercepted and read in the Legislature by

MacDonald, "I must prepare a speech of some kind. This is not hard right now because I happen to have a pretty good speech already prepared by someone else that I have permission to use and can adapt to suit my needs."

"Having that," Knox continued, "I can go off on any tangent — just any tangent at all. Therefore I could, without any trouble, take great pains to scorch Donald MacDonald, especially as the speech refers to industry in our riding anyway."

Knox wrote that he had to weigh "whether I might embarrass you or the department of health any further by whatever publicity it [the speech] might get or by whatever further remarks might be made by Donald MacDonald or his ilk."

Knox, who would lose his riding to a Liberal in 1967, was dismissed by MacDonald as a "Tory lackey of industry."

In the northwestern Ontario town of Dryden similar conditions, if not intrigues, prevailed. In the Dryden chemical plant mercury vapor billowed from the mercury-cell process installed in 1962, clinging to ceilings, walls and floors. Men were periodically tested for mercury in their urine and pulled off the job when levels climbed too high. Occasionally, physical signs developed before the levels reached the maximum. Some men suffered bleeding gums and nervous twitches. Some lost hair and were quick to come down with ailments.

"The early symptoms, of course, were bleeding gums," a former Dryden worker would later reveal. "It affected your nervous system to a certain extent. You would have twitches you didn't have before. Your arms and what-not. But mostly it was the bleeding of the gums."

"They liked to put it down as an industrial hazard rather than a compensable thing. The practice was to remove you from the area until your count went down. Put you outside. They really didn't care what you did, so long as you were out of the area until your count went down. A lot of us sat on the rocks to get a suntan."

The worker said he just assumed his health was being safeguarded by the company. But when the disorders became apparent around 1964 and 1965, employees began to question whether management really "gave a damn". "It's kinda hard to control mercury," the worker conceded. "I'd say the company did try, to the extent of their knowledge. But I don't think they knew anything about what was going to happen. Nobody knew that much about it. . . . They didn't do their research. It was as if management were saying 'This is the thing [mercury] that we are going to use, and we're going to use it. If it goes out the sewer, it goes out the sewer. That's our loss.'" The worker concluded that "they didn't want to lose too much, but at that time I don't think health was as big a factor as the expense."

Years later, company officials would deny that mercury posed any significant occupational health problem. Only "two or three" ever had to be compensated for health damage caused by mercury, according to Loren Chudy, a public relations officer with the Dryden mill's parent company, Reed Paper Limited.

Chudy emphasized that workers inside the plant were exposed only to inorganic mercury, not methyl mercury. "And what the medical people generally indicate is that mercury can be flushed out of the body fairly readily if it's not a steady intake. As a general procedure in any plant where there may be a substance that's causally harmful, the procedure in our company, and all companies that we are aware of, is to take that person out until the levels go down and then, if he wants, to go back."

Robert W. Billingsley, who became Reed Paper's president in 1973, acknowledged the medical threat posed by mercury, but also stressed the difference between the two forms of mercury. "It was methyl mercury we were not aware of," he said, "the conversion of the mercury in the bottom of lakes and into the food system through the fish . . ." Billingsley said that from "the old 'Mad Hatter's Disease' of the eighteenth and nineteenth centuries it was known that mercury could have harmful effects on people. Within a plant environment you can always have very strict rules for any kind of toxic chemicals. That goes for even the trace elements we all need to live. You have to watch it and you test."

"But that was elemental mercury, and we had to watch for it coming off from the air as well as water. I'm not aware of the details of what we were doing in the sixties. I know what we've been doing in the seventies, and it's a fairly routine kind of practice, and we've had no problems that I'm aware of in the last many, many years."

If nothing else, their comments illustrated the casual manner in which modern industry approached the use of potentially hazardous chemicals. The medical risks associated with elemental mercury were not reduced by the discovery of methyl mercury. The symptoms of mercury poisoning from either form are similar and can be equally critical, although methyl mercury is admittedly more deadly because it is readily absorbed into the bloodstream.

The chemical industries of Dryden and Sarnia were of particular concern to Norvald Fimreite. They dumped their effluent into rivers whose waters supported both sport and commercial fishing, providing potentially poisoned food for humans. But he was also interested in the broader environmental effects of mercury, particularly on wildlife.

London was a good spot for his work. A quiet, white-collar city of about two hundred thousand, it was central to both farm and industrial operations — in the heart of Ontario's agricultural breadbasket and equidistant from the factories ringing Toronto and Detroit. A leisurely drive away were three of the Great Lakes — Huron, Erie and Ontario — the largest body of fresh water in the world. The region supported healthy fisheries, and migratory birds stopped to feed on flights to and from the boreal forests of the Canadian shield.

Fimreite believed the largest quantities of mercury and mercury compounds were logically being lost in the area of greatest industrial concentration, in the southern Great Lakes basin of Ontario and the St. Lawrence River valley of Quebec. Ontario and Quebec could probably account for two-thirds of all mercury used — and lost — in Canada. Conversely, the place to look for mercury in agriculture was where farming dominated the environment, on the prairies.

Money was no problem. With the security of his federal grant, the young ecologist set off in a rented camper in the summer of 1968 for western Canada, armed with a rifle and a licence to shoot any species of bird he desired for testing. Prairie farmers were unnerved by the sudden appearance of this brazen eastern scientist who was blasting birds out of the sky. "He damn near got shot himself," said George, his supervising professor. The birds were frozen and sent to a laboratory for analysis. Excessive mercury levels were found, presumably from mercury-treated seed grain.

Fimreite's studies of mercury levels in pheasants and partridges led the government of Alberta to close the hunting seasons on the birds, fearful of the possible effects of consuming these birds on humans. He said the mercury could probably be traced to the fungicide Panogen, which had created similar problems in Scandinavia.

That summer he also had fish collected in British Columbia and from the Ottawa River, near chlor-alkali plants and pulp mills. The readings recorded during the fall and winter confirmed his suspicions. Fish from the Ottawa showed mercury levels of two parts per million. In a grebe, a fish-eating bird, found by a lake near the mercury-producing Cominco mine in B.C., a reading of seventeen ppm was registered. Chickens and game birds on the prairies commonly revealed levels of five ppm. All exceeded the .5 ppm federal standard.

As returns came in from his mail survey of chlor-alkali industries, Fimreite decided to go public with some of his early findings. At a seminar at the University of Western Ontario on February 28, 1969, he warned that "in this area we must anticipate mercury contamination. The aquatic ecosystems are most likely to be contaminated, with the highest amounts of mercury appearing at the ends of food chains in animals such as large predacious fish, fish-eating birds and mammals. . . ." He was saying that significant sections of Ontario might be contaminated, fish poisoned and humans endangered.

While his words were largely unheard beyond the university walls, the message grated on the nerves of some members of the audience — particularly officials of the Ontario Water Resources Commission (OWRC), the provincial agency (now known as the water management branch of the environment ministry), whose job it was to conduct pollution-control surveillance. A few months earlier they had lifted soil samples from the bottom of the St. Clair River as part of a broad water-quality survey of the Chemical Valley. The cores had been analyzed for several pollutants, but not mercury. Despite Minamata's deadly experience, no one on this side of the Pacific Ocean had been aware that mercury discharged into rivers and lakes could be harmful, let alone lethal.

Following Fimreite's alert, however, OWRC scientists returned to the lab to take another look at the samples. The technology for conducting mercury analyses in Canada was primitive, but after much

I am not aware that mercury compounds pose a pollution problem in Ontario, nevertheless I will be pleased to institute inquiries to find out if this is the case. *George Kerr*

effort, the OWRC laboratory in Toronto made the samples reveal their evidence of mercury; some readings were as high as fifty parts per million.

Fimreite continued to collect fish samples, but on the advice of his supervisor he also began experimenting on red-tailed hawks and pheasants under controlled conditions at the Niska Waterfowl Research Station near Guelph. Dr. George wanted Fimreite to demonstrate how mercury accumulated in the wildfowl. The student raised chickens on seed laced with mercury fungicide and fed them to the hawks. Twenty-seven succumbed after their livers malfunctioned under the assault of mercury levels of seventeen to twenty ppm. The pheasants reacted similarly.

Scientists with the OWRC meanwhile were seeking further information on the extent of mercury contamination in the St. Clair River and Lake St. Clair. They began poking probes into the sediments upstream and downstream from the Dow plant. The findings were startling. From samples above the plant, they recorded trace amounts of the element. But from cores lifted from the riverbed immediately below the plant, the scientists discovered the sediment was saturated with as much as 1,400 ppm of mercury, nearly as great a concentration as that found below the Chisso plant in Japan.

The mercury problem remained very much a matter for scientific concern and study through the spring and summer of 1969, but in June of that year the first rumblings of political discontent were heard when Fred Burr, the environment critic for the New Democratic party, asked then Energy and Resources

Minister George Kerr about possible contamination in Ontario.

The NDP member from Windsor asked: "In view of the abandoning of the use of mercury compounds in Japanese agriculture and the banning of mercury fungicides in Sweden and recent awareness of the many industrial uses of mercury that result in air and water pollution, will the minister investigate the seriousness of this recently recognized pollutant as it affects Ontario?"

Kerr replied: "I am not aware that mercury compounds pose a pollution problem in Ontario, nevertheless I will be pleased to institute inquiries to find out if this is the case."

Burr later revealed he had no real reason to suspect that Canada had a serious mercury problem. He had simply read about the sad experiences of Minamata and Sweden in the popular press. "I just wondered if it was happening in Sweden and Minamata, whether it was happening here. I just wanted to know whether our people had been keeping up with the news and, by and large, I discovered they hadn't. I suppose nobody was given the task to keep an eye open. Perhaps they were too engrossed in shuffling paper," he suggested.

With the discovery of the massive mercury discharge from the Dow plant, officers of the OWRC moved to introduce a program under which Dow could reduce its mercury losses. Meanwhile, the first halting steps were taken to determine whether aquatic life had been affected by the pollutant in the river and lake. Acknowledging Fimreite as the only available expert, the OWRC asked him if he would

My advisors tell me that the mercury
which is found in our streams
is not of such an extent that we should be concerned.
George Kerr

participate in a sampling program. The commission would net the fish, dissect inch-square cubes of fleshy tissue and make them available to Fimreite. He could send his samples to a sophisticated laboratory at the University of California at Berkeley. The OWRC would conduct its own analyses at the Toronto lab.

In October of 1969, officials of the commission braved choppy waves and chilly pre-winter blasts to net twenty-two fish from the river — pickerel, suckers, rock bass, shad. Each was cut up, weighed, tagged and sent away.

On October 27, the energy and resources minister told the Legislature that mercury was in fact being used in some Ontario paper mills but, said George Kerr, "the amount of mercury used is very small. We have no specific method in Ontario of specifically testing for mercury, because of the problems in carrying out an analysis on such minute quantities."

By November, Fred Burr was impatient for answers about the state of environmental affairs in Ontario and once again asked Kerr to provide them. Following repeated questioning, Kerr revealed that ministerial orders had been issued on plants in northern and southern Ontario to cease mercury discharges. Later, an Opposition member was ruled out of order when he asked the PC cabinet minister if he could "give us assurance at this time that the levels are not dangerous."

Burr was inflamed by the government's procrastination. Kerr was either ill-advised or not advised at all on the extent of the problem. Burr complained on November 19 that he had "been trying to get the government to become concerned about mercury pollution ever since last May." Burr asked Kerr to "just state that he feels a sense of urgency in the matter of mercury pollution." In a response that would characterize the government's attitude in the years ahead, Kerr replied: "My advisors tell me that the mercury which is found in our streams is not of such an extent that we should be concerned." His comment was made despite the fact that the OWRC still did not know how much mercury might be found in the fish of the St. Clair.

In early January of 1970, the OWRC completed its studies of the fish samples taken from the river three months earlier. Two of the fish had mercury levels exceeding twenty parts per million, most were in the teens. The readings were up to forty times the acceptable level for human consumption set by the World Health Organization and the federal government, but the commission was still concerned about the accuracy of its testing methods and waited to hear from Fimreite. It would be kept waiting. Fimreite received his results in March. They were as high as the OWRC's, but rather than compare notes he reported his findings to the Canadian Wildlife Service, which alerted federal authorities in the fisheries department.

The OWRC first learned of Fimreite's results when one of its scientists, conducting door-to-door interviews with Chemical Valley residents on their opinions about water quality in the area, was told by a housewife that the federal government had ordered the fishery on Lake St. Clair closed because of mercury in the fish. Officials inside the OWRC were miffed over Fimreite's going to the wildlife service without consulting them. But Fimreite said he was annoyed by the attitude demonstrated by the OWRC and other provincial authorities toward the crisis. "I felt they were too busy finding excuses for not having done anything until the disclosure of high levels in the fish," the young scientist said. "Much could have been done if they had simply admitted that they were not aware of the problem."

Dime Jubenville and his boys were still enjoying the celebration of a bountiful fishing trip when they received a telephone call at the Lighthouse Hotel at about seven-thirty.

"Dime?"

"Yes."

"Have you shipped your fish yet?"

"No, but it's in the truck."

"Well, I guess you'll have to take it off. We have to hold them for tests for mercury."

The word went out around the lake. Lawrence Drouillard, a sixty-three-year-old sturgeon fisherman, was told to lay up his gear, unaware that the order signalled an early retirement. Pat Hamilton, a young father, a fisherman since the age of fourteen when his father died, put away his boat and like many others began filling out unemployment insurance forms. As the days and weeks of idleness passed, the fishermen of Lake St. Clair slowly found other jobs, none of which really appealed to them. Some took work in factories, others hired on as farm workers. Still others began pumping gas at service stations in the district.

The closure of Lake St. Clair was total. The western basin of Lake Erie was also affected. It created a public furor, and Fimreite found himself in a spotlight cast by the press.

Some members of the zoology department at the University of Western Ontario, complained privately about the public attention being paid to the graduate student. They felt his work was being prejudiced by public debate before being subjected to proper academic review. Torn between the unrelenting demands of academic research and a compulsion to report his dramatic findings to an increasingly pollution-conscious public, Fimreite opted to talk to reporters and risk upsetting his colleagues.

His supervising professor, Dr. George, quit the project. "We had a division," he said. "He felt he was capable of carrying on without my advice, so I refused to have any more to do with him." George complained that Fimreite, though timid, was strong-willed and liked the limelight. "He would listen to what we had to suggest and then he would do it his own way. He became very independent of any supervision from the university. He became consumed by the publicity and, in doing so, didn't do a real good scientific study, what we would consider good science."

Fimreite claimed the rift between himself and George was caused primarily because he had had two supervisors in the early stages of his research. George had filled in for William Holsworth when Holsworth made his field trip to Africa, and wanted

Fimreite to spend more time on the controlled experiments with pheasants. Tensions built between them. When Holsworth returned from Africa, he resumed the responsibility for supervising Fimreite, and defended his student.

"Although the release of mercury into the waterways has been going on for five to twenty years," Holsworth stated in a letter of reference in 1971, "it was not until Mr. Fimreite's ecological approach to the problem was made public that industry and the governments became concerned . . . It is abundantly clear that Mr. Fimreite's study has been one of the major events in directing the path of public concern, industrial responsibility and government action towards a better, healthier environment. Mr. Fimreite has handled the publicity of this situation very capably, maintaining the position of a concerned scientist."

Fimreite would be awarded his doctoral degree after making some revisions to his thesis. He joined an engineering consulting firm that specialized in assessing the impact of industrial development on the environment. His works would be published in a number of scientific journals and eventually he would return to his native Norway, to a teaching position at the University of Tromso.

Meanwhile, Dime Jubenville and the others pulled their boats from the lake, unable to market the fish that had provided a living for generations of Lake St. Clair fishermen.

"I want to go back," Dime said. "I've got a lot of miles on me. But it's a way of life. It's a heritage that's been in our family for over a hundred years. It's a way of life we understand."

3

The Politics of Pollution

The pollution crisis that forced the closing of the Lake St. Clair fisheries raised a monumental row in the Ontario Legislature at Queen's Park in Toronto. Any member of Premier John Robarts' Progressive Conservative government who poked his head above the rim of the political trench in April 1970, was a fair target, and George Kerr was the most obvious target of them all.

As energy and resources minister, the man responsible for the purity, or lack of it, of the province's water bodies, Kerr was accused of everything from simple incompetence to outright criminal neglect. But over the years on the front lines, he had developed a thick skin and had become something of an expert at deflecting the slings and arrows of political warfare.

A lawyer by profession and eternal optimist by necessity, the veteran politician from Burlington, a growing dormitory town between Hamilton and Toronto, regularly downplayed the threat of pollution. To those who were angered by the death of Lake Erie, he vowed to drink a glass of water from the lake within five years as evidence of his government's ability to revive it. To those who protested that Burlington Bay had been turned into a cesspool by Hamilton industries, he promised to swim in it one day as proof that the Progressive Conservative government was at work, as always.

For most current residents of Ontario, there had never been anything but a Progressive Conservative government. The Liberals had fallen from grace in fractious disarray in 1943 and showed no signs of regaining power. Their efforts were complicated by the increasing popularity of a third party, the union-supported, pro-labor New Democratic party. The two opposition parties had to share the anti-government vote, but the Liberals had more representatives elected to the legislature, and were the official Opposition party, so the Progressive Conservatives, or Tories, had remained in power since the war, relatively secure on the ship of state, which rocked only when big waves struck it.

In the years following the Second World War, pollution was not an important issue. There were other matters to occupy the politicians, practical bread and butter matters such as the provision of jobs for returning veterans and the creation of a peacetime economy, one which could continue to prosper now that the production of war machinery no longer provided an impetus. The early popularity of the Progressive Conservatives in the post-war years could be traced as much to their dedication to economic expansion as to the disintegration of the Liberal party as a viable political force. Tories pledged themselves to the expansion of industry and extension of public services, especially education.

To accomplish their objectives, they proposed to fully exploit the province's natural resources, and that meant opening new mines, granting logging rights to companies over vast tracts of forest, offering tax breaks to industries of all kinds and developing an electrical network to provide sufficient power to meet the increased demands.

The Conservatives largely achieved their goals. As the province headed into the 1960s, Ontario could boast an educational system generally ranked among the world's best, one that produced an ever-increasing number of university graduates. Ontario Hydro was a giant in power production and the province was linked by an efficient network of modern highways. Health care had been greatly improved and social and labor legislation introduced to give Ontario residents the highest living standard in the country, almost equal to the prosperity of their richer U.S. neighbors.

But the economy hummed to a tune played by industry. Industry was allowed great concessions because the Progressive Conservative party was convinced that what was good for industry was good for people. The discharge of waste and its subsequent impact on the environment was seen as an unfortunate necessity of an industrialized society. But popular attitudes had undergone a drastic change since these post-war years. By the sixties there was a rapidly increasing undercurrent of public opinion that we were paying a high price for the material benefits of modern technology, indeed that matters were out of hand in North America and society was placing itself at profound risk. In the 1960s, the anti-pollution movement had been growing on fears raised by United States ecologists such as Paul Ehrlich, Barry Commoner and Rachel Carson, the author of *Silent Spring*, a powerful condemnation of society's growing dependence on chemicals, particularly DDT. By 1970 people of all ages were profoundly worried and wanted their politicians to act.

"I am being told that my world is so polluted

**I am hoping that as the water becomes fresher,
the fish will become healthier.
Let us put it that way.** *George Kerr*

that I will not even have a chance to die a natural death," a university student told an international pollution conference held in Hamilton, Ontario, earlier that year. He told of reading "that I will sink in garbage before I get a chance to die – and then will likely have to be buried in it anyway.

"Adults today cry at youth for destroying what is good because that will only lead to chaos. Perhaps chaos would be better than the hell we've got now."

Increasingly, these fears were expressed to politicians, sometimes in the confusing jargon used by scientists, sometimes in simple statements by schoolboys. During the debate on the government's handling of the mercury crisis, Jack Stokes, the New Democrat member for the northern riding of Thunder Bay, shared one such letter with the Legislature. "I am a boy of eleven who is worried about pollution of all kinds," the youngster had written him. "I try myself to stop it, but I alone am not good enough. I am not worried about now, but about when I am 22. What is going to happen to me and all others?"

Public pessimism had become so widespread and deeply felt that both opposition parties joined in the attack on George Kerr and the large band of Tories seated across the red-carpeted aisle of the legislative chamber from them. Robert Nixon, leader of the provincial Liberal party in 1970 led the assault.

"We in this province – in fact on this continent – are on the verge of an ecological disaster," the Opposition Leader warned. "This particular case of mercury poisoning simply shows that with the best attempts and with all the funds we are able to

provide, we are still caught by surprise in circumstances of this type."

Energy and Resources Minister Kerr, of course, defended his policies. "I feel," said Kerr, "that if we can eliminate the source of the mercury pollution that, by time . . . any fish that are contaminated will lose that contamination, and also more fish will not be contaminated. I am hoping that as the water becomes fresher, the fish will become healthier; let us put it that way."

His response to the mercury crisis clearly rested more on hope than on reality. He said the polluted rivers and lakes would be dredged and, in a matter of weeks, perhaps fifteen or twenty, the waterways and the fish would purge themselves of the poison. Indeed, Rene Brunelle, the minister responsible for lands and forests, flatly forecast a complete recovery within three or four months.

"Once the source of the contamination has been removed in those areas the fish would be edible within a matter of somewhere between seventeen to twenty weeks," he stated, although conveniently failing to provide scientific support for his heady proclamation.

Brunelle, who gained entry to the provincial cabinet more by virtue of representing the politically isolated north than for his intellectual prowess, must have been dreaming. Government ministers surely would not lie. In any case, a technological solution to the problem did not exist. Scientists were fully aware that mercury compounds were insoluble in water, almost indestructible. Dredging, even if such an enormous financial undertaking were possible,

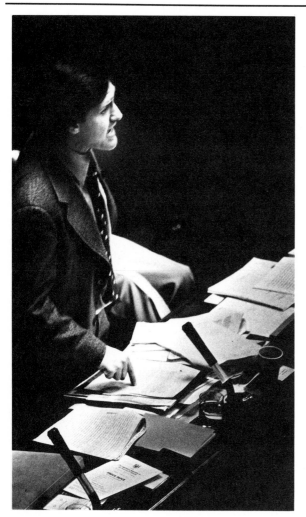

Stephen Lewis, Ontario Legislature, 1976.

would simply dislodge the mercury from the bottom mud and set it adrift to relocate. Mercury ingested by fish would eventually find its way back to the bottom when the fish died — a never-ending poisonous cycle.

Dr. William Holsworth, Norvald Fimreite's supervisor at the University of Western Ontario, was openly pessimistic about the ability of the St. Clair River and Lake St. Clair, or any other body of water, to recover in this century from the environmental damage caused by mercury. He warned that "if the fishermen are waiting around until they can fish again in this area, they might be very old men before that time. For the foreseeable future, everything we know about the problem suggests it will remain contaminated for decades. Whether it's centuries or not, we have no way of knowing. It will be at least thirty or forty years. There is no indication it will be less."

Nonetheless, Rene Brunelle and George Kerr clung to their unfounded belief that the waterways would swiftly recover. They promised dredging as the panacea to the pollution sickness. In fact, the government would later learn, even if a mechanical cleanup were possible, the cost would be astronomical, perhaps one hundred million dollars.

The April, 1970, debate had followed on the heels of Kerr's March 31st announcement that mercury levels of fish seized from Lake St. Clair fishermen had been found to exceed the .5 ppm federal standard for export and human consumption. With his political experience, he knew the furor the announcement could trigger and had tried to ward off his critics by undercutting them. He said samples analyzed during the winter were "not alarming" and, besides, the federal standard was probably overly protective of a people whose fish consumption was relatively low by international standards. But, he stressed, he was discharging his responsibility to the people of Ontario and had issued ministerial orders to end the flow of mercury into rivers and streams around the province.

Eight pulp and paper mills were using mercury in the papermaking process, but three had already discontinued its use, Kerr reported to the Legislature. The remaining five, he said, were ordered to stop using mercury by April 15, two weeks away. Five chlor-alkali plants "where work is not so far advanced" had been told to eliminate mercury loss by May 1.

When Kerr added that "the discharge of mercury into waterways poses no danger to drinking water or to swimmers," Liberals and New Democrats roared their disapproval of the minister's incredible defense. The two opposition parties said prosecution of the polluters should begin immediately. Why, they asked Kerr, did the Ontario Water Resources Commission not order Dow Chemical last fall to stop discharging mercury, rather than waiting until the poison was detected in the fish of the St. Clair.

"This is when we immediately started working with Dow Chemical to reduce that to where it is now, almost nil," the minister replied. "It was at that point [last fall] that OWRC moved in and steps were taken to reduce that waste."

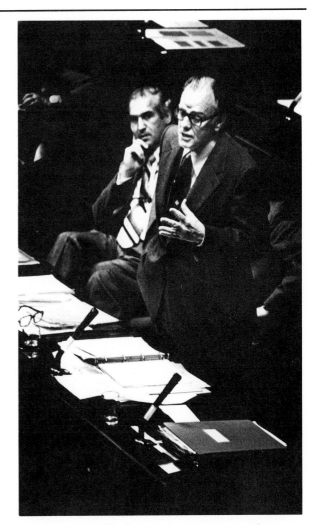

Leo Bernier (seated) and George Kerr, Ontario Legislature, 1976.

I drew your attention to the fact . . . in 1964.
What was done from 1964 on?
Donald MacDonald

"That is not so," argued Stephen Lewis, the New Democrat from the Toronto-area riding of Scarborough West. "That is just not so." Lewis's good memory would become greatly respected in the years to come, as leader of the New Democrats, especially when this party became the official Opposition in 1975.

Kerr countered Lewis by saying that it was "very difficult to establish any form of contamination by just analyzing the water or the effluent. It is only through checking the fish that we are able to establish any danger area from contamination or pollution. This has only been established very recently."

"I drew your attention to the fact . . . Dow Chemical was polluting waters with mercury poison in 1964," NDP leader Donald MacDonald noted. "What was done from 1964 on?" His question went unanswered.

"Am I right," Lewis asked, "that the minister earlier said that OWRC began working with Dow in the fall of 1969?"

"Yes."

"Well, then, why was nothing done until the poisoning was found and then, suddenly, within ten days, Dow was able to terminate the mercury discharge?"

"Something was done," insisted Kerr.

"Nothing was done," Lewis maintained. "The OWRC sat on its hands for six months."

Kerr kept his composure, and went back to the possibilities of dredging.

"It is quite possible," he insisted, "that there could be some form of dredging. A great deal of this mercury compound sits at the bottom of the lake. Some of the bottom fish accumulate this mercury and then, subsequently, they are gobbled up by fish such as walleye. So it may be, by some sort of dredging, or cleaning, or scraping the bottom of the lake, we can eliminate what accumulation of mercury is there. That, coupled with prohibiting discharge of mercury into the lake, seem to be the only two remedies we have."

He blamed his government's delay in acting on the general lack of technology in Canada that would determine the biological effects of mercury on the environment.

"We just did not have the facilities here to make a detailed analysis of fish," he explained. "The fish that were taken from the lake apparently were sent to California for analysis, and this takes some months. It was only in the last couple of months that the findings were made known . . . .

"Our first results of the analysis of these fish was in January of this year," he continued, "so we certainly have acted, I think, as quickly as possible. The whole idea, the whole question of mercury in fish and the methods of analysis and everything was not perfected to any degree. We did not have the expertise here."

"Except in Japan and Sweden," interjected Nixon, the Liberal leader.

"Yes, well, we knew what happened in Sweden, but then . . . "

Dryden mill, Wabigoon River, 1976.

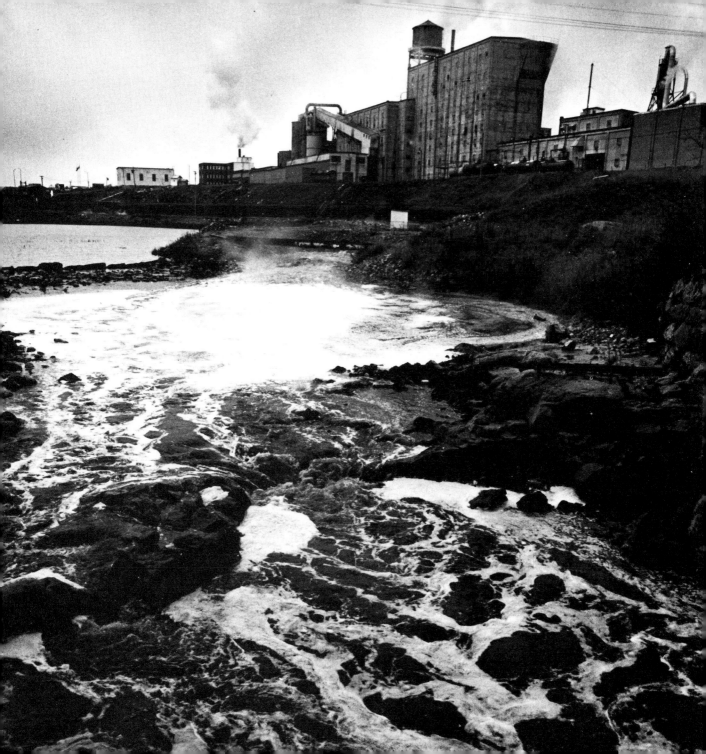

**Because it was lying on the bottom of the river
did not mean it was polluting the water.
Our responsibility is over water.**

John Root

"You knew months ago," Lewis pointed out.

"In my view," said Nixon, "the responsibility [for the pollution] lies primarily with the provincial government and the minister has been derelict in his duties in not acting with dispatch." Nixon called attention to a newspaper interview in which an OWRC official had said Kerr had not been provided with an early alert on the mercury problem. "We do not inform the minister of every little pollution problem we see," the official had told the press.

'I can see under certain circumstances," said the Liberal leader, "that this approach would certainly be a reasonable one. But when mercury is found to be in the sediment of one of the Great Lakes . . . and even those of us who are not dealing with this on a day-to-day basis have been aware of the disastrous results of similar pollution in Japan and Sweden, it is difficult to understand why an official in the minister's department would consider this a 'little pollution problem'."

Intelligent debate ended when John Root, a Tory member for the rural riding of Wellington-Dufferin, rose to defend the role of the OWRC in the sorry episode. Root was vice-chairman of the commission. "The mercury, as far as we knew, was lying in the sediment on the bottom," Root explained as he entered the debate, "and there are many things lying on the bottom of lakes and rivers."

"How do you suppose it got there?" asked MacDonald.

"Our responsibility," Root continued, "is to help municipalities get adequate supplies of good potable water and bring pollution under control wherever we find pollution existing. And as soon as we found — "

"You found it and you did nothing!" charged Nixon.

"Because it was lying on the bottom of the river did not mean it was polluting the water," replied Root. "Our responsibility is over water."

With that, the vice-chairman of the OWRC tried to limit the commission's responsibility. Presumably, what was needed in Ontario was an Ontario Sediments Control Agency.

Opposition members persisted in their attack on Kerr and the government, persisted to the extent of accusing the minister of "criminal neglect" in his failure to recognize the problem earlier and move vigorously to correct it.

Finally provoked beyond what he considered reasonable, Kerr shouted back at his antagonists: "Industry is the polluter in this case not the government. Remember that." His defiance set off a wave of catcalls. "Industry is the thief," he repeated. "We are the policemen . . . "

More hoots of derision.

"It is obvious," said Kerr in the confusion, "that Lake St. Clair has been polluted for twenty years. It is obvious — "

From across the chamber, his critics yelled that it was logical to assume, therefore, that government should have acted twenty years ago.

"All right," Kerr argued, "but who knew about it first. Who knew about it first? Industry knew about it, and if they have got any conscience at all, they will start cleaning up. We will do our part, but we are sick and tired of trying to be Sherlock Holmes . . ."

Again, laughter and shouts filled the House.

"We will continue to play detective," Kerr continued, "but we want to think that we are dealing with responsible people who are just as concerned as we are about the environment of this province."

Kerr promised that the victims of pollution would be compensated, and cited legal action as one of the "drastic remedies" open to the government to recover damages to people downstream from the polluting industries. But his pledge was dismissed as so much idle rhetoric.

"If I may pick on the analogy that the minister has introduced," said MacDonald, "the problem is that the policemen have been in league with the thieves down through the years. That is the problem."

The debate dragged on, and on, and in the course of the melee it was disclosed that the Ontario companies ordered to prevent any further loss of mercury in their operations were Beaver Wood Fibre, Thorold; Spruce Falls Power and Paper, Kapuskasing; Canadian Johns-Manville, North Bay; Strathcona Paper Company, Strathcona; Domtar, Cornwall; Dow Chemical, Sarnia and Thunder Bay; Canadian Industries Limited, Hamilton and Cornwall; American Can Company, Marathon; and Dryden Chemical Company, Dryden.

If nothing else, the debate revealed Dow as the plant under major political attack. But even as the debate continued, authorities were poring over fish samples from other regions, particularly the waters downriver from the pulp and paper operations at Dryden in northwestern Ontario.

There was cause for alarm.

4

The Case of Ball Lake Lodge

As Ball Lake emerged from its winter slumber there were only subtle signs that the summer of 1970 would be different from the other happy, prosperous summers of the past quarter-century. Spirits were high. None anticipated the disaster that loomed.

Almost as the ice retreated from the docks and sandy beach, Indian men and women appeared from Grassy Narrows, Andy Keewatin and Joe Loon and the others, anxious for fishing to begin.

In Kenora, Marion Lamm rushed completion of her extraordinary shopping expedition, accumulating the supplies needed to fete a summer of hungry anglers — steaks to soda pop, pickles to popcorn. A white-knuckle flyer despite husband Barney's love for and dependence on airplanes, Marion would grudgingly make only one flight into Ball Lake in May, another out at season's end in October, a hundred-mile round trip of nervousness aboard a bucking Beaver float-plane. She wanted nothing of mid-season shuttles to and from stores.

Everyone worked confidently toward the season opening, despite disquieting rumbles about pollution in the river system. Men lugged boats to the water's edge, or tinkered with troublesome outboard motors in the boathouse. Women scurried about the laundry and kitchen, restocking shelves, taking inventories, while teams swept winter cobwebs from cabins dotting the site. Barney and his pilots made repeated flights in with material and the stocks piled up on the docks.

The Lamms loved Ball Lake Lodge for many reasons. They had arrived here in 1946 as honeymooners and their five beautiful daughters, like the lodge, had grown to maturity by the lake. Memorabilia filled the place. Here, too, was where their fortune was made, enabling Barney to establish a veritable northern air force, 33 bush planes, Cessnas, Beavers, Norsemen, a Grumman Goose or two, even a trusty old DC3. He used the planes to fly guests into the lodge, or cargo into points north, making a fortune along the way. The lodge, if a price could be placed on it, was worth about one and a half million dollars. And the planes, well, around Kenora it was acknowledged that Barney Lamm was well-heeled and, therefore, fairly influential.

"Ball Lake," said Marion, "is our whole life." The May rush was on to make it ready for the arrival of the first guests, due to arrive in just a few days.

Chicago business executives were regulars among the guests, coming individually, with their wives or in chummy charter groups, happily trading their pinstripes for jeans, windbreakers and rumpled old hats. Others hailed from New York and Los Angeles, and Canadian cities such as Toronto and Montreal. There had been visits by celebrities, too — newsman Edward R. Murrow, golfers Sam Snead and Ben Hogan, singer Frances Langford and actor Robert Taylor. Teamster boss Jimmy Hoffa showed up one summer to escape Detroit's union wars and vowed to return. Hoffa, now believed dead, had joked with Andy Keewatin, the chief fishing guide. "When I get back here next year, we'll start a guide's union," he had promised.

Barney's Ball Lake Lodge was clearly a misnomer, a name that lost its appropriateness soon after newlyweds Barney and Marion arrived from Minnesota after purchasing the "lodge", as it was then called. In the years that followed, it grew on cash provided by a burgeoning leisuretime society to become a hamlet, a unique wilderness retreat among birch, spruce, poplars and towering Norway pines — "You're not supposed to cut those," Barney always emphasized. "They belong to the Queen."

The central lodge was rapidly expanded and the first cabin, their honeymoon haven, was soon joined by others, built along paths paved with pine needles. Twenty-five cabins, all built of hand-hewn logs, eventually occupied the acreage. The Lamms and the Indian staff built a boathouse and a freezer, where meat was stored along with the fish which the sportsmen would take home with them; fine, firm fillets, specially packaged for the paying customers. They built a laundry, a store, a residence for the young Indian girls who served as waitresses and kitchen help, and a hall for meetings and dances. There was even a chapel, where visiting clergy of all denominations were invited to conduct services, accompanied by one of the Lamm girls on the Hammond organ. Everything was powered by a diesel generator, an enormous, immaculately maintained piece of machinery that had been hauled through the bush to illuminate the summertime community.

Barney adapted a golf cart to serve as a fire engine and drew great pleasure in occasionally putting on a fire chief's hat and racing through the camp to lend a little excitement to routine relaxation. It was one of the "gimmicks" used by the shrewd outdoor businessman to keep his guests amused and anxious to return. Another little luxury was a self-serve beauty salon, with curlers, dryers and appropriate accessories, for those women guests who needed to maintain their city facade even in this wilderness setting.

When the weather turned sour, there were pool and tennis tables, always crowded, under Tiffany lamps. Or the idled fishermen could play poker in a games room decorated with trophies of an African safari made by Barney in 1965.

"After your first day," the advertising literature told the sportsman, "you will know this is the vacation you've been looking for."

The Lamms worked hard to attract and satisfy their guests. Each January, they would leave hometown Kenora to make the circuit of sports shows through the northern United States, adding new customers to the regular, steady trade. At the peak of most seasons prior to 1970, as many as one hundred visitors were at Ball Lake, and up to seventy-five persons from Grassy Narrows were employed there. In autumn the lodge also offered facilities for hunters of ducks, deer and moose. But fishermen clearly paid the freight.

The ads boasted: "Barney's. Where the hunting and fishing exceed your wildest dream. Our guides will take you to great sport, whether it's northern pike, muskie, lake trout, walleye or bass. You say what you want and you'll get it . . . They are all here in abundance."

The boast was largely accurate and well received. There were other camps along the Wabi-goon and English rivers, seventeen in all, but none was as profitable as the lodge at Ball Lake. Barney Lamm was indisputably the king of camp operators. He even owned a 10 per cent share of Minaki Lodge, a big resort down the English-Wabigoon chain, beyond the Whitedog Indian reserve on the Winnipeg River. Controlling interest of Minaki was held by an American businessman.

Barney employed some white guides, vacationing college students, but his business thrived in large measure with the help of the Ojibways from Grassy, men who lived their lives by the water, instinctively knowledgeable in the movements and habits of the fish beneath the surface, fish whose size and courage were legend. (The Indians had been noticing an increasing number of fish in recent years floating to the surface, but it was a phenomenon they did not dwell on.) The people of Grassy benefited by tying their fortunes to Barney's Ball Lake Lodge. His success paid their wages. Guides were paid fourteen dollars a day, plus their room and board, and could expect substantial tips if they followed Barney's lead and pampered the wealthy guests. A summer at Ball Lake was fulfilling in many ways.

Many of the guides brought their families and lived in cabins separate from the main area. The youngsters would earn spending money at odd jobs, such as camp cleanup or catching minnows for bait. Almost without exception, boys spending their summers here, such as Matthew Beaver, aspired to be guides like their fathers. They were encouraged to learn the intricacies of fishing and the fine arts of filleting and cooking, to man an outboard and to anticipate changing weather.

Matthew, a good-looking youngster who easily won friends with his infectious smile, learned his lessons well and became one of the favorite guides of the regular guests. They would often ask for him when making their reservations and it was not uncommon for him to receive a hundred-dollar gratuity from a group of appreciative visitors, additional reward for his long days and careful attention.

Matthew usually rose shortly after six each morning to bring coffee to his guests' cabin by six-thirty. His boat was ready to push off at seven-thirty, bound for secret spots along the English River, deep holes where lazy trout hid, or shallows where stealthy northern pike preyed on frogs. In his boat would be a box containing all the ingredients needed to transform the fish into a gourmet meal, to be enjoyed in the quiet splendor of a shoreline clearing.

A shore lunch was the stuff of memories — campfire, pork and beans, spaghetti, bread, strawberry jam, coffee, a box of beer and frypan loaded with freshly caught fish that had been dipped in egg, covered in crushed cornflakes and sizzled in hot bacon grease. Lunch alone could absorb three hours. Fish caught in the afternoon were usually destined for the freezer and the trip back to the city.

At night, as the guests relaxed in the luxury of the lodge's spacious lounge or played poker in the back room, the Indian guides would retreat to their cabins, where they might sip some home brew. The Lamms tolerated no nonsense from their staff when

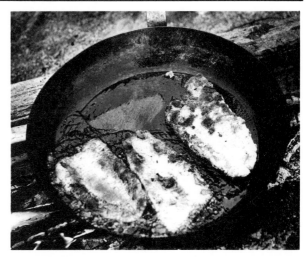

A shore lunch of fresh caught fish.

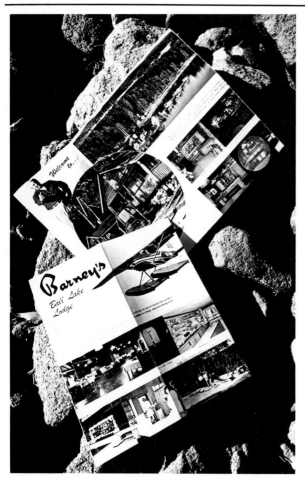

As things used to be at Ball Lake Lodge.

it came to drinking. Anyone creating a disturbance by dipping too deeply into the brew pot could expect to be punished, much like an errant schoolboy, with the loss of privileges. One of the first privileges to go, if a guide was troublesome, was the Saturday night dance, a favored affair among the staff.

"Alcohol is a problem with the Indians," Marion Lamm recognized. "Certainly it is a problem. But in the twenty-five years we operated, we never had occasion to call the police. There was liquor at Ball Lake. There was liquor all the time. The American tourists always had liquor and took beer out in the boats. But nobody ever beat anybody up. We just didn't have that problem."

Every two weeks, on payday, Barney would hold a staff meeting to discuss the operation of the lodge, little things that might have cropped up since the last payday. He would offer his guides a beer, "a little free beer, so everybody would come."

"We used to discuss what the guests wanted. I used to preach that this was the best goddamn camp and the reason is that the staff is the best. Indians are good workers, but you can't push them. We used to talk about how you can't push anybody and I used the description of the rope. 'Look, take this rope. You can pull it, but you can't push it.' They would get a kick out of those sorts of things and laugh about it."

Barney knew how to get the most from his native staff. If one of the men was assigned the menial task of pumping out the floats of one of the planes and a guest was within hearing distance,

Mercury completely changed our way of life.

Marion Lamm

Barney would make a point of asking if the plane was okay for use.

"The next morning, you would see them pumping the floats and having everything ready. This was our psychology, like lining up the boats on the beach. I'd say, 'now get them straight. Hey, there's one out of line,' and they'd get them all lined up and stand there and grin. The next night they'd have every boat lined up just so. We used to have a lot of fun doing these things with them."

The boss also provided a full summer stock of retail goods to be sold by the Ojibways in their independently operated shop. He wrote off the cost. He was a soft touch for an emergency loan and often made his planes available for mercy missions. Perhaps it was paternalistic, but Barney's "psychology" yielded a growth of jobs and profits, and was endorsed by a staff whose loyalty was almost total.

Once, when a broken oil line downed Barney's plane on a remote lake overnight, a group of guides set out, unannounced, and found him at dawn before a search party could be organized. In the late 1950s, at a special ceremony at Ball Lake, residents of bands across the district made him an honorary Ojibway chief.

"Ball Lake wasn't just a livelihood," explained Marion. "It provided us with a very good living, and for our children, but we also loved the place. We liked the outdoors, the people we dealt with, the affiliation we had with our employees. The relationships we had gave us pleasure. We couldn't have built Ball Lake and it wouldn't have been successful without them. Mercury completely changed our way of life."

The Lamms first learned about mercury from Walter Booey. A long-time camp operator down the Wabigoon River from Dryden, he told his fellow camp operators at a meeting in April that mercury had been found in unusually high levels in the fish of Clay Lake. Barney and Marion felt no personal threat. The source of the pollution was at least eighty miles away. So, when the pollution alert was issued by the provincial government a week before guests were to arrive at Ball Lake in mid-May, they were shocked and confused. Plans for the season were thrown into disarray as politicians debated the issue at Queen's Park.

Mercury was a dangerous pollutant, health authorities stated, a potentially deadly poison. Mercury levels in fish at Ball Lake were not exceptionally high, but worrisome enough to close commercial fishing and place restrictions on the camps. The politicians assured the operators the mercury discharge up the river system had been stopped and it was just a matter of time before the waters and the fish purged themselves, perhaps fifteen or twenty weeks.

The Lamms decided to close the lodge at Ball Lake temporarily rather than expose their guests and guides to the risk of poison, regardless how minor. They invited their customers to attend Minaki Lodge, on the Winnipeg. Fifty-four anglers registered at Minaki, but within days the rumors had spread even there that the pollution had hit the Winnipeg River. Barney pestered the government in Toronto for answers, telephoning Rene Brunelle,

Ball Lake Lodge, 1976 season.

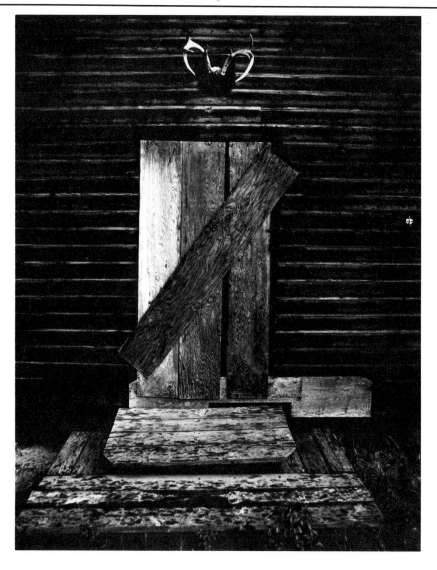

the Ontario minister for lands and forests. Brunelle confirmed the rumors. Barney told his guests the fish was not safe and broke out beef and pork chops to feed them for the remaining three or four days of their vacation.

The government groped for answers to the dilemma, then side-stepped the issue, suggesting that camp operators could continue to offer "fish for fun." In a telegram received by the Lamms May 15, Brunelle said health authorities "recommend that anglers return their catches to the water except for trophies."

The Lamms knew that to inform their guests that shore lunches had to be eliminated, that they could not eat the fish, was to doom the lodge to bankruptcy. It would only be inviting a flood of cancellations. Without hesitation they dismissed the idea and turned to the moral questions posed by the temptation to remain open and bluff it out until the pollution threat passed.

"Can we have Joe Loon go out and eat the fish? We don't have to eat them. But can we send the boats out with the guides? Can we put ourselves in the position where we could be sued?"

Some operators, with less capital to fall back on, decided to risk it, but the Lamms said no. They decided to close down the lodge at Ball Lake. It would, after all, only be for one season, fifteen or twenty weeks, during which time they could gather information on mercury pollution — what it was, where it came from, how it hurt people. Their decision, they were convinced, was right; but it carried terrible consequences for themselves and the people of Grassy Narrows.

The guides were sent home and Barney and Marion faced the task of notifying all of the sports fishermen who had reservations and still planned to come to Ball Lake. They were sent a bulletin:

"We regret to announce that due to mercury pollution in some lakes in the territorial waters of the district of Kenora, Barney's Ball Lake Lodge is not open. The lodge is ready to operate, but we do not feel we can accept any guests until such time as the mercury pollution in the water and fish is at a safe level for human consumption . . . .

"My business has been built on being honest and frank with my guests. I have been advised by the authorities that at the present time the fish from these waters should not be eaten. Therefore, under the present circumstances, I do not feel that you could have a safe and enjoyable trip. The source of the pollution has been stopped and I am hoping that it won't be long before all our valued guests will be able to return for another memorable fishing trip to Barney's."

At the top of the bulletin, they sketched the caricature of a fish. The fish optimistically told the anglers "I am sick, but recovering."

5

Fishing for Fun

When the Dryden is dumping all the junk in the water, that's why it makes mercury. And it flows over our lakes. And when the people catch the fish and eat lots, they get very sick.

Please don't eat fish. It can destroy your life.

—Children's posters,
Grassy Narrows School. 1975

The native staff returned home to Grassy Narrows; Barney and Marion Lamm headed for Dryden. They did not understand how mercury was used in industry. They wanted to learn, first hand, and with the instinct and naivete of amateur detectives they went to the source. It was late May and the air of the town was warm and pungent with the unmistakable, unpleasant odor of the mill, a smell even some Dryden natives were unable to ignore. The Lamms were struck by the size of the chemical and paper mill complex. It was situated on a plateau overlooking the once-wild Wabigoon River. Its tall stacks and billowy white clouds, which dropped residue indiscriminately on homes, cars, people, everything downwind, dominated the low-slung downtown skyline.

The outfall pipe from the pulp and paper mill was clearly visible alongside the heavily travelled highway. It spewed forth its effluent. The river frothed and vapor rose in the air. Between 1962 and 1970 the company had lost about 20,000 pounds of mercury to the Wabigoon. Tons of solid wastes — bark, woodfiber, dirt and chemicals — were also discharged daily into the river. Methylation of the mercury was facilitated by the presence of the raw

A Grassy Narrows home, 1975.

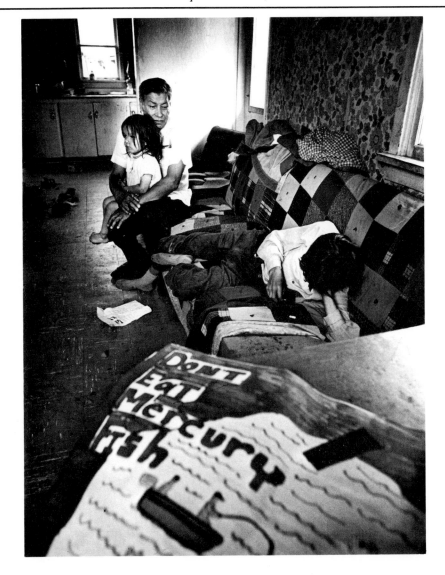

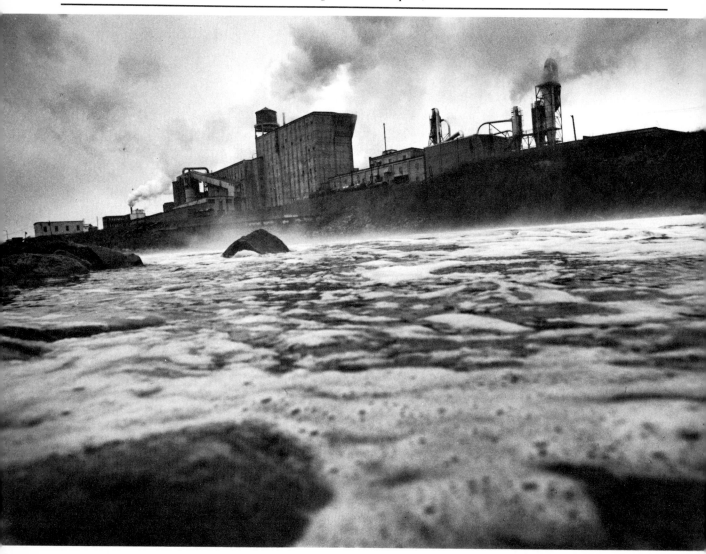

The Wabigoon River at Dryden , 1976.

Fishing boats, 1975.

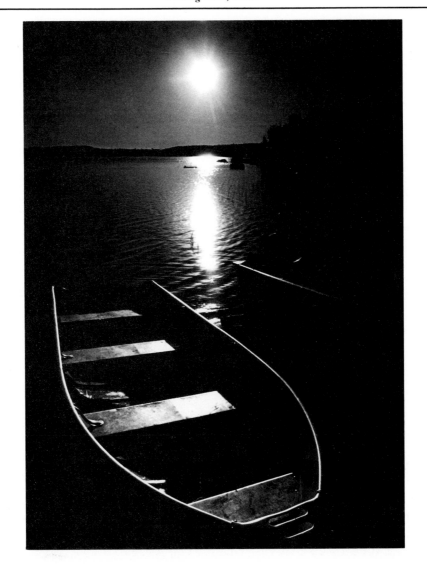

Contaminated catch, 1976.

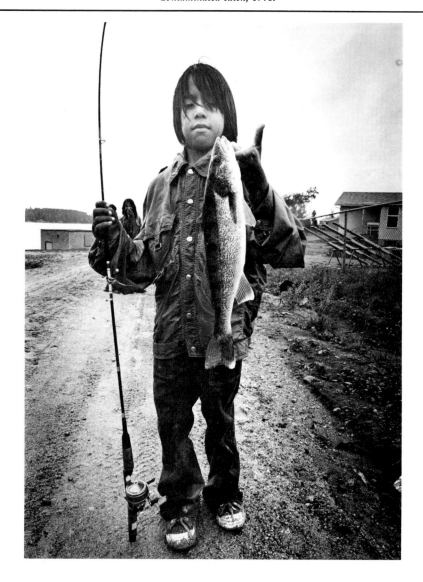

Contaminated catch, 1976.

industrial sewage, which created the anaerobic conditions necessary for the transformation to take place.

The scene seemed strangely out of place, a contradiction, an ugly sore on an otherwise attractive northern community. The irony was that without this industry, which provided a livelihood for roughly six thousand men, women and children, the community could not exist. Although Dryden was dependent on the plants of Dryden Chemical and Dryden Pulp and Paper for its economic survival, it was also strategically situated to serve a flourishing tourist and recreation trade.

"This is a friendly town in the center of a beautiful lakeland area," said the literature. "We hope you will have time to stay a while and enjoy it."

Mayor George Rowat was quick to explain to skeptical southerners that residents really enjoyed living in Dryden, despite the sweet smell of industrial success. "The thing you people don't understand," he would say, "is that we don't live here because we have to. We live here because we want to."

But certainly the force that made the choice possible was the mill. Built in 1913, it employed roughly a thousand persons, practically one person from every family in town. Another 500 or 600 worked in the woodlands. The money from its monthly million-dollar payroll powered commerce and made luxuries possible. And municipal politicians were always aware that the mill provided almost 40 per cent of the town's tax base.

Few of the employees had ever met their bosses.

Oh, they knew their superiors by sight and often by their first name. T. S. (Tom) Jones, the manager of the operations, was a familiar presence in town. But the owners were largely anonymous to the hundreds of families who depended on their benevolence and business acumen. The Dryden mill was part of an international conglomerate, a child of the Anglo-Canadian Pulp and Paper Company, itself a branch of the powerful Reed Group of companies, with headquarters in Britain. Tom Jones was also a vice-president of Anglo-Canadian Pulp and Paper, Reed's Canadian wing.

Reed International Limited was pretty much a power unto itself, a vast organization which drew its strength from profitable forest exploitation. Unlike its political counterpart, this British empire was expanding, extending its corporate interests into forty or more foreign countries. By 1976, it would employ as many as one hundred thousand workers in pursuit of a billion-dollar annual revenue.

The Reed organization, though vast and complex, was exceedingly efficient. Powered by investment from private stockholders, and sometimes government subsidies and tax breaks, it loomed large in such diversified fields as mining, fashions, publishing and hydro-electric power development. But its chief interest was wood. Its subsidiaries produced everything from cardboard cartons to furniture, newsprint, gummed tapes, wallpapers, toilet paper, and more.

Unannounced, the Lamms arrived at the gate of the Dryden chemical plant and were met by a watchman who readily agreed to show them the

We have caught it
before there has been any real danger to human beings....
Jack Davis

mercury cell. He explained how the mercury performed as a kind of floating electrode in a salty brine to produce chlorine and caustic soda, how it was flushed free and sometimes lost to the sewer. The tour was brief but informative, and for the first time the Lamms were able to relate the words "mercury pollution" to something they had actually seen.

The amateur detectives, however, would soon discover that further information would be more difficult to gather. They quickly learned that not everyone was as anxious to know the intimate details of mercury in the environment. They discovered that the provincial government was all too willing to clutter the route to facts with red tape. The government refused to release mercury levels of fish in Ball Lake, claiming the studies were ongoing and incomplete. Officials would say only that levels exceeded health standards. Little help or enlightenment could be expected from Ottawa either. The federal government's attitude to the problem was reflected in a statement made by Environment Minister Jack Davis, who claimed credit for catching the problem before people could be hurt.

"We have caught it before there has been any real danger to human beings," he announced. "Once spotted, we have closed the fishery. Either that or we have bought up all the fish and had them destroyed. Nothing has escaped the watchful eye of our federal fisheries inspection service — a service which is regarded the world over as tops so far as fish quality and public health is concerned."

The Lamms clearly had to look elsewhere to find answers to the questions they wanted answered. They barraged experts with mail inquiries for information and gathered whatever literature they could find on mercury pollution. They even attended a seminar at a Michigan university, where they learned that, despite the heady forecasts of George Kerr and Rene Brunelle, waterways contaminated by the element could remain so for a century because the technology did not exist to purge the pollutant.

In June, they hired Norvald Fimreite to conduct an independent survey downriver from Dryden. They wanted to scientifically document the extent of the damage and to satisfy themselves that the decision to close the lodge at Ball Lake was the correct one. The survey required a second trip to Dryden, so the Lamms and Fimreite returned to the town. But their access to the plant was prevented by a fence. Why, they wondered, are people trying to hide the facts?

Armed with bottles for taking water and sediment samples, the trio walked along the banks of the Wabigoon, lifting evidence and marking labels. Workmen along the river saw Marion dunking for water and shouted: "I don't think you should drink that."

From Clay Lake Fimreite netted a variety of species and bagged waterfowl along the shores, repeating the tedious exercise downriver, in restful coves and open stretches, meticulously tagging the wildlife for later identification. After weeks of collecting, he had 510 samples of fish, birds and animals.

The results of his investigations were even more devastating than those of the St. Clair basin in Southern Ontario. One large northern pike, found floating on the surface of Clay Lake, yielded a mercury reading of 27.8 parts per million. Walleye ran to 19.6 ppm, a reading equal to those of fish found in Minamata Bay. Numerous fish taken along the watercourse to Ball Lake revealed readings in their teens, thirty to forty times the safe level. The Wabigoon and English river systems were clearly suffering from severe mercury contamination.

Fimreite's public statements about his findings created a local stir among tourists and lodge operators. In August, he was told by the district provincial forester that his permit to collect wildlife for scientific research had been revoked, because he had not submitted a listing of animals taken. Fimreite claimed the list was not required until the end of the year and noted that by a strange coincidence, the permit was revoked immediately after he had publicly criticized the wildlife branch of the Ontario department of lands and forests for its handling of the mercury problem.

Fimreite said the action was typical of a number of government agencies. "They not only refused to co-operate, but even tried to stop my investigations in northwestern Ontario. . . . Regarding the health authorities, I suggested to them on several occasions that investigations be undertaken to reveal any effects on those who had consumed the heavily contaminated fish in large quantities — Indians in northwestern Ontario for example. They hesitated in commencing such investigations."

Only after Fimreite had turned over his findings to the Lamms did the Ontario government confirm that its samples had revealed similar readings. But in public, at least, the provincial government clung to its position that the crisis was temporary. Sport fishermen were told the fishing was as good as ever, but, please, do not eat the fish for a while in these ten lakes: Clay, Ball, Indian, Grassy Narrows, Lount, Separation, Umfreville, Tetu, Swan and Eaglenest. Literature circulated by the Ontario department of tourism advised against shore lunches and take-home stringers but stressed how "the angler may still catch and keep that 'one for the wall' since trophy fishing is not prohibited."

From the beginning, Lands and Forests Minister Brunelle's Fish for Fun program was patently unworkable in an area where fishing was not only a pastime of tourists with lots of money to spend, but a way of life for Indians. The government was attempting to discharge its responsibility by telling people to fish and eat their catches at their own risk. Fish for Fun also helped deflect claims of loss of camp operators forced to close because of the pollution. Ultimately, the maneuver victimized the camp operators as well as the Indians. While health authorities warned against eating fish from the polluted waters, other departments of government were saying that fishing could continue, knowing full well that no angler would spend hundreds of dollars for a northern vacation if he had to throw his fish back into the water. Meanwhile, the commercial fishermen of Grassy Narrows and guides idled by the closure of Barney's Ball Lake Lodge had lost

**We'll be flying through the whole area
and the minister has even suggested
he may go for a swim in Clay Lake.**

Leo Bernier

income and therefore were increasingly dependent on fish from the polluted waters to feed their families. Brunelle's department of lands and forests distributed and posted Fish for Fun signs, each bearing the symbol of fish in a frypan crossed with an 'X' and a warning that fish should not be eaten due to mercury pollution. But the signs did not stand for long.

Some camp operators could not understand why customers should be scared away and business damaged, since the problem was only "temporary". Indian guides who were still employed were offered a bottle of whiskey for each sign destroyed, and the government made no effort to replace them. Guides were told to prepare and eat shore lunches and keep their mouths shut about mercury. The crisis would pass.

The Lamms sensed that a wedge was being driven between themselves and the other operators. They spoke openly and often against the continued operation of the camps. They spread the information they had gathered about mercury and this upset the government. Rather than alert the public and visiting anglers to the dangers of mercury, Energy and Resources Minister George Kerr and Leo Bernier, the Progressive Conservative member for Kenora, launched a counter-campaign.

In August of 1970, Kerr went on an open-line radio program in Kenora. He said he was touring the district to explain to people what had actually happened, "in case they are getting wrong information about it, or exaggerated information about it."

"I think it was unnecessary for any camp oper-

ator ... to close right down at the opening of the season," Kerr said. "You know, a lot of people are happy to come up here to Fish for Fun and there are also hundreds and hundreds of areas in northwestern Ontario where the fishing is still very good, very excellent, and they are not too hard to reach."

"By closing a camp down and making a great to-do about it and publishing information that isn't exactly accurate and may be a little emotional, this has hurt the whole industry in this area."

While accusing the Lamms of distortions and emotional exaggerations, the minister went on to promise, once again, that dredging would solve the problem and commercial fishing would soon resume. "If this is minimized," he said, "we are hoping by next year we won't have the high levels of mercury contamination from these certain areas that have been banned this summer."

Bernier, along to lend support and feed questions to the minister, applauded the news and asked: "Mr. Kerr, I wonder if you could report if there have been any reported ill effects to humans from mercury pollution in the province of Ontario?"

"No," Kerr replied to the planted question. "We know of no situation where any individual has become sick as the result of mercury contamination."

Bernier told the area radio audience that later in the day he and Kerr would be making an aerial inspection tour of the Winnipeg and English River systems. "We'll be flying through the whole area," the local Tory stressed, "and the minister has even suggested he may even go for a swim in Clay Lake." The suggestion had a familiar ring to it.

Bernier had a significant stake in keeping the camps open. A northerner himself, the forty-two-year-old former bush pilot was anxious to extend a political career begun in 1966. The son of a merchant in the small town of Hudson, forty miles northeast of Dryden, Bernier prided himself on understanding the problems of small businessmen, and he often voiced opinions which identified him with corporate interests. In any case, he knew the north country and was pledged to its development. Both Dryden and Kenora were included in his riding and he strove to minimize the crisis in the public's mind, lest business be affected and votes be lost. He wanted to see northern Ontario share some of the south's industrial wealth and that meant keeping industry and tourism on a healthy footing.

In the Legislature in November of 1970, Bernier was attracted by easy solutions. He complained that the .5 ppm federal standard for mercury was too low and should be lifted to 1.0 ppm, thus enabling fishing bans to be lifted on some of the less affected lakes. And he attacked "prophets of doom and the sensation seekers."

"Man has begun to overpower the environment, both with his ingenuity and sheer numbers," he conceded. "At the same time, however, we face the danger of being overwhelmed by pollution hysteria and falling victim to pollution of the mind. I do not advocate minimizing the dangers of pollution or the necessity to clean up the air, soil and water.

"However, our approach must be rational and collective. The roles of government and industry and the individual are very much interrelated and interdependent ones in the war we must wage to rescue our environment. Responsibility for pollution control measures and their cost will have to be shared."

Behind the rhetoric was a conviction that health authorities were overreacting to the pollution problem. Bernier claimed he had eaten fish from the chain for years, and nothing had happened to him. By his words and actions he encouraged the delusions of the worried camp operators.

The operators were in a tough position. With large amounts of capital at risk, most were prepared to do whatever was required to get over the rough period which, they had been assured by the politicians, would be short. The Northern Ontario Tourist Outfitters Association maintained a strict silence on the issue. No literature on mercury pollution was prepared and camp owners along the polluted chain said not a word on the subject. Kenora's tourist offices co-operated, speaking of mercury only when visitors raised the topic, then responding with ridicule. In Dryden, a sick joke made the rounds, that the way to get rid of mercury was to hang the fish by their tails in a freezer and, when the temperature dropped low enough, cut their heads off.

The government encouraged the camp owners to downplay the problem. It was anxious to avoid emotional claims for compensation. "Our policy," Bernier would later confirm, "is that there will be no compensation for industrial pollution. The polluter is responsible and the courts are open to individuals to take on the polluter. The thing (about compensation) is, where do you stop? It could be endless in terms of industrial pollution damage — the lead plants in Toronto, sulphur damage in the Sudbury area, smoke damage, respiratory diseases. It would be endless." He justified the continued sports fishing by concluding, "They are only up there for a week or two at a time."

Colin Myles, operator of Hook's Camp on Separation Lake, which employed about twenty-five Indian guides, wanted to believe the Fish for Fun program could work. But he would not lie to his guests. At the beginning of the 1970 season, he and his wife had sent telegrams to everyone who had made a reservation, telling them that fish from the ten lakes downriver from Dryden should not be eaten. They said the fish from uncontaminated lakes would be provided for shore lunches and repeated the department of tourism's publicity pitch that 'trophy' fish could be kept. The Myleses received a flood of cancellations. "Although you can furnish fish from other waters," one angler wrote, "we believe that one of the thrills of being your guest is to catch and eat our own fish."

With supplies already purchased and advance publicity funds spent, the Myleses limped through the summer with a skeleton staff and scarcely a quarter of their regular business. Then they closed their doors, forever, at an estimated loss of about $300,000.

One unsympathetic tourist official would later blame the failure of the Separation Lake camp on poor management. "While we realize your operation is in the center of the area in which the contamination is prevalent," he wrote the Myleses, "we point out to you the successful efforts of others in similar situations over the past year . . . surely you can learn from their experience that despite the adverse publicity regarding the contamination problem, with perseverance and good operation, your resort could continue to operate."

"We feel cheated," said Mrs. Myles. "It wasn't our fault. We've had no help at all to recover anything. It's been a complete loss and we are too deeply in debt to start over again. We knew there was no way to continue operating at Separation Lake unless the fish were safe to eat, or we had to lie to our customers. It was one or the other."

Colin Myles added, "Our business has been jeopardized through the fault of the polluter and the polluter should be held responsible. But, unfortunately we do not think we can afford to take this to court."

Barney Lamm, however, had the resources and launched a legal action against the Dryden Chemical Company and the Dryden Pulp and Paper Company, claiming $3.7 million in lost land, fixed assets and anticipated profits. By March 1977, the suit was still unresolved.

The Lamms and the Myleses remained convinced they were right in telling their customers all the facts available and in closing their camps. But they gained no sympathy from Bernier, who turned his back on the maverick operators. He claimed they were overreacting, and in that claim he chose to ignore the opinions of health authorities.

"I have no hesitation in stating as my opinion

It's not only the person who eats the fish who might be affected, but the unborn offspring.
Dr. R. B. Sutherland

that the fish from these waters should not be eaten," Dr. R. B. Sutherland, chief of the Ontario ministry of health's health studies service, said in an interview.

"I don't think it will do any harm if a person has the odd meal of fish with more than .5 ppm," he said. "I think the problem basically is that to eat more than that isn't necessarily going to affect the health of the person eating the fish — but we don't know what possible genetic effects there might be.

"There were some infants affected in Japan, so there is a sort of grey area where we have to be careful. It's not only the person who eats the fish who might be affected, but the unborn offspring."

Dr. Sutherland said the .5 ppm level established as the ceiling for human consumption appeared realistic, given the lack of contradictory evidence. "I don't think we want to play around with this kind of potential hazard." But Bernier turned logic on its head and decided that "this problem of mercury contamination of certain of our waters is the result of new knowledge that is still imprecise."

The 1970 season was a disaster. Tourism was off throughout the district, and at Grassy Narrows the people were left confused after visits by health authorities who drew blood samples, snipped hair, checked eyes and asked them to stand on one leg. The results of the tests were withheld, but they were told not to eat any more fish. Just off their shores, they watched American anglers enjoying the harvest of English River country. What kind of madness was this? True, there were fewer sport fishermen on the lake this summer, their numbers depleted by

fears the whole of northwestern Ontario was polluted. Some camp operators reported trade was off as much as 60 per cent, but that was little consolation to the Indians.

Fearing further losses in 1971, operators on the polluted waterways banded together and appealed to the provincial government for aid. They called themselves the Fish for Fun operators and they asked the government to either declare the fish safe to eat, introduce a subsidy program to cover losses, or close the polluted waters and buy the camps, enabling them to relocate on clean lakes. The last option, they estimated, would cost $4.3 million.

"We are desperate," they stated in a brief presented to the Ontario premier and his cabinet. "No longer can we continue to operate. This is not the result of our mismanagement. This disaster occurred through no fault of our own and it was not an act of God.

"Government must provide us with urgent and immediate assistance. We have not voiced our dilemma to the news media. We are responsible enough to keep silent, until you have a final chance to act. Our 'demands' are not those of a militant organization, but the rational demands of small businessmen in big trouble. We are about to lose everything!"

The government ruled out the proposal to close the system and buy the camps, figuring it would smack of compensation. Instead, it offered a loan program to prop up the operators until more information could be gathered on mercury, and better times returned. A similar loan program was offered to idled commercial fishermen on Lake St. Clair. But the government was simply buying time, not solutions, and the camp operators were left to struggle into another season under the shadow of mercury poisoning.

Down on Baptiste Creek, Dime Jubenville was having his own hard times. "The reality," said Dime, "is just beginning to set in. It wasn't too bad last year. There was a lot of confusion and you couldn't keep your mind on it. But now — on a mild day like this — this is the best kind of a day to bring them in."

"It's the season, you know. There's a season for everything. There's a season for golf and duck hunting. And this is the fishing season. This is it, and it's becoming a reality. It's like an accidental death — like someone dying and then, all of a sudden, you realize he's not coming home anymore."

The comments of the veteran Lake St. Clair fisherman had the same ring as the Myles', a bitterness and helplessness over what had happened, a realization that everything they had was gone.

"What we have here is nothing today," Dime complained. "We were cut off for no offence. Dow committed an offence against the taxpayer and all they've done is reduce the flow of mercury. We're out of business and Dow Chemical is still reaping a profit."

"We've never asked the government for a nickel in the past. If the going got tough, we tightened our belt. And if things went well, we might put an extra window in the house. But we feel we've been wronged — by somebody."

Government, meanwhile, ordered more studies, more tests, and assigned task forces to the job of assessing the situation. Recommendations were made and promptly shelved for more study.

At Grassy, the people were becoming poorer and poorer. Welfare payments which in 1969 ran to $2,400 a month were on their way to the $12,100 mark. The social consequences of that fact were in large measure ignored by provincial politicians who, when pressed, only repeated that no medical evidence of Minamata Disease had yet been discovered.

Meanwhile, the federal government poked away at its own studies. Fish were lifted from Clay Lake and sent to laboratories in Ottawa, where they were fed to cats in controlled doses. As the mercury levels escalated, the cats went into the dance of death so familiar to Japanese scientists. The people of Grassy Narrows, and beyond them in Whitedog, were not informed of the frightful experiments.

In February, 1971, the Progressive Conservatives picked a new leader to succeed retiring Premier John Robarts. The choice was Brampton lawyer William Grenville Davis, the education minister in the Robarts administration. Davis promised a fresh approach to government and placed environmental protection high on his list of priorities. One of his first cabinet appointments was Bernier, to the portfolio of mines and northern affairs. Bernier would go on to the ministry of natural resources, where he would become the primary target of pollution critics.

Davis was swift off the blocks in setting the tone of his regime. With great fanfare, the young premier

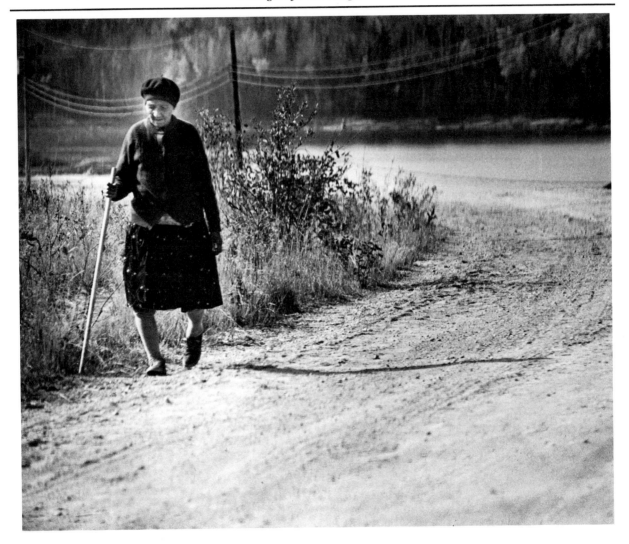

A changed life, new village, 1976.

Walk to the only water tap, 1976

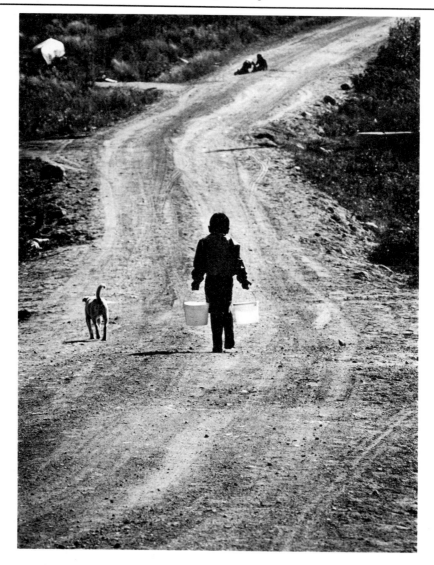

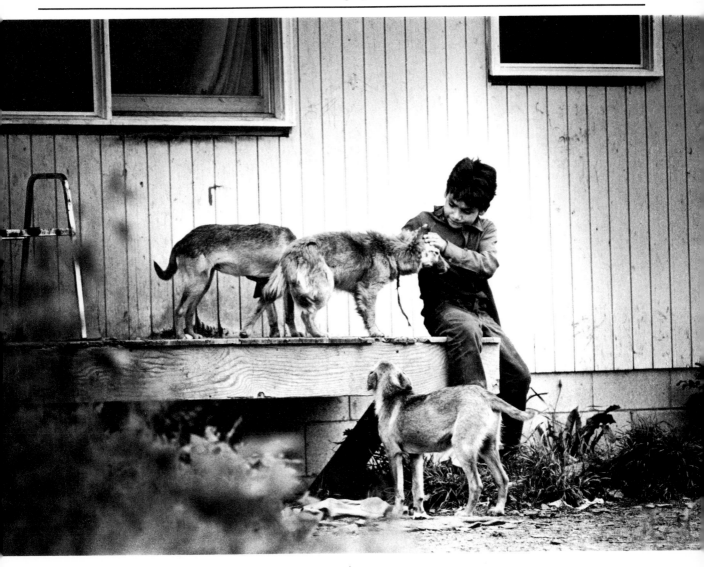

No one has come in and explained to us what levels we have.
Bill Fobister

called a press conference March 15 to announce that the government was launching an unprecedented twenty-five-million-dollar law suit against Dow Chemical and its American parent firm. If a cleanup of the St. Clair basin could not be achieved, a further ten million dollars would be sought in damages.

The premier said the case would guide the government in its dealings with other polluting companies, but Liberals and New Democrats assessed the action as a grandstand play to win votes in an anticipated autumn election, which the Tories won handily. Years later, the assessment would gain credence as the government watched unconcerned as the action languished in the courts.

By the summer of 1971, the people of Grassy Narrows had become dependent on welfare. Those who wanted employment were forced to move off the reserve, and many did, including Marcel Pahpasay, who took his family down the road to the railroad community of Jones. Rosy Pahpasay was pregnant again, for the fourteenth time; but this child would never breathe the air of English River country.

"The baby never moved," said Marcel. "It was just like air blowing her up, because the baby was sick. I wish I was more educated. I could tell you what really happened. She just had the baby and it was dead." The Pahpasays buried their child in an unmarked grave. Many residents of Grassy were worried about their health, but drinking had become such a problem that it was difficult to tell whether they were truly suffering from mercury or simply too much alcohol. Symptoms were similar and white doctors tended to attribute speech defects and lack of balance to chronic alcoholism.

In the meantime, government was jealously guarding its findings of mercury in the people of Grassy Narrows, fearful that the readings might be misinterpreted and prompt unfounded panic. No diagnosis of Minamata Disease had yet been made. But, then, the authorities were not looking very hard. Tests were inconclusive, done in the spring when fish consumption was down. No effort was made to conduct an epidemiological survey, a mass testing program to document the physiological impact of mercury on the entire reserve.

When Andy Keewatin, then chief of the band, appealed for information on tests already completed, he was told simply that some samples showed blood levels of seventy parts per billion, the measurement commonly used in blood samplings. Some victims of mercury poisoning in Japan recorded readings of 200 ppb, although most were higher.

G. J. Stopps, hired as an environmental health consultant in the Ontario ministry of health, told the people of Grassy Narrows by letter: "This is the sort of result we expected, but the results were also not high enough to suggest that anyone in your band was suffering from mercury."

His response enraged Bill Fobister, the band's young administrator. "No one has come in and explained to us what levels we have," he complained. "They don't even have any measures on how much mercury would harm us. They haven't informed us what levels are dangerous. I don't think

**It appears
it has been strictly a case of putting dollars before health,
not only for tourists, but also local citizens.**

Marion Lamm

---

they know what is the danger point."

In Kenora, the Lamms experienced a similar frustration and growing hostility toward their stubborn campaign to keep mercury in the news.

At first, former friends would simply ignore them on the street, cross to the other side or snub them outright. Then the resentment took a more disturbing form as their antagonists began making threats against the family by telephone. One Friday night a drunk former guide from Ball Lake chased Marion across the street, yelling "Your head is full of mercury. I'll fix it!"

The attitude also surfaced in sober conversation. A local businessman, annoyed by the drop in trade he attributed to the Lamms' outspoken grievances, snapped at Marion, "One thing I know for damn sure, it wasn't for humanitarian reasons you closed."

"What other reason could there be?" Marion replied. "I can't understand you. We had nothing to gain and everything to lose."

Rumors of all forms circulated around town, the most popular being that Barney Lamm's operation at Ball Lake had been in trouble and he was using the Indians to win a bundle of needed cash from the paper mill, a rumor he flatly denied.

Marion wanted Barney to move, but he refused. "We're not going to run away from it," he said. "We are right." If anything, he was more convinced than ever that government had become a pawn of industry and people must be recompensed.

Evidence of the devastation mercury could cause was steadily growing. In New Mexico, the children of a poor farm family were blinded and crippled

when they ate pork raised on a mercury-treated grain. The United States government banned the sale of swordfish after people who had eaten small amounts of the fish showed symptoms of mercury poisoning. And news of the worst mercury disaster in history was just beginning to filter out of Iraq.

Mercury-treated seed grain was distributed to farmers in broad reaches of Iraq in September 1971. The seed was meant for planting, but two years of famine led many to use the grain for food. Thousands were poisoned by their own homemade bread.

Anxious to cover up the tragedy, the Iraqi government belatedly imposed a news blackout. It would be years before the extent of the catastrophe would be known — 6,530 recorded hospital admissions, 459 deaths. The toll, however, was much greater than the official record. Statistics for the period revealed 3,264 deaths more than had occurred in the same period the year before.

The Lamms wanted the Canadian public to have access to all information on the subject of mercury. In April 1972, as Kenora once again prepared for another troubled tourist season, they appealed to the municipal council.

"It has been quite obvious for nearly two years that, in Kenora, any information regarding mercury pollution has been suppressed by radio, newspaper, word of mouth, etc.," said Marion Lamm. "It has not only been suppressed, the seriousness of the situation has been ridiculed and erroneous rumors started about anyone that talked about mercury poisoning . . .

"It appears it has been strictly a case of putting

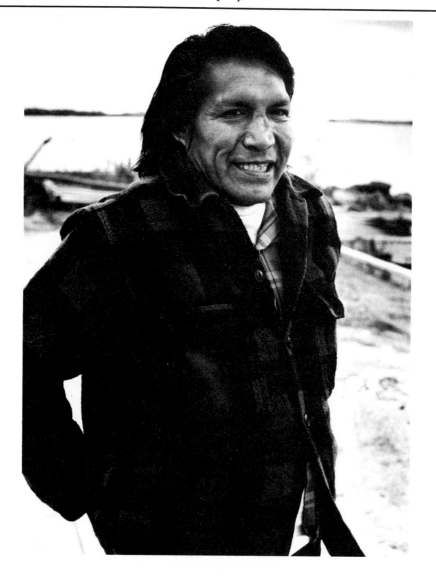

dollars before health, not only for tourists, but also local citizens. The attitude seems to be 'If we don't talk about it, the tourists won't know that we have extremely high levels of mercury in the fish in certain areas of the Kenora District.' Unfortunately, mercury does not go away . . ."

"I would like to make it clear what our feelings are on this. The saying is 'Put up or shut up.' We have put up, a million-dollar business and twenty years of hard work, and we have no intention of shutting up."

Rosy Pahpasay once more gave birth to a child, this time in the comfort and care of a hospital in Kenora. It was a boy, born six weeks premature. He barely survived. They named him Keith and took him home to Grassy Narrows. He was much like all the other Pahpasay children, except perhaps a little more sickly. He had trouble holding his bottle and when he was ill, he took longer than most to recover.

During one illness, the Pahpasays were sufficiently worried to take him to town, where he was confined to hospital. The nurses discovered Keith was blind and gradually the severity of his brain damage became known. He was just a year old.

As one season yielded to the next, the people of Grassy Narrows tried to live normal lives, despite the mounting unemployment and increasing tendency of jobless men and troubled women to bring alcohol onto the reserve. Drunkenness and strife were spreading.

Still, what normal patterns remained were pursued and as the air turned brisk in the early autumn of 1972, Tom Strong took his wife and children by canoe up the English River to harvest the wild rice.

Tom Strong was a hardy man, a trapper and guide and, therefore, a heavy fish eater. At forty-two, he had seen many seasons and experienced much of the contentment of English River country. But times had turned sour. His people were in disarray and he, too, was suffering. Lately he had been losing weight, his speech was becoming slurred, and he had been bothered by slight pains in his chest.

The rice waved heavy in the wind and fall colors flashed in the trees as the Strongs set up their camp in a quiet cove called A.H. Bay. They pitched their tent, gathered wood for the campfire and prepared to bed down for the night. It was then that Tom Strong was stricken.

He rose to his feet and gripped his chest as pain coursed through his body. He cried out, staggered forward through the flap of the tent, and fell dead to the ground.

6

What Do You Have to Make Us Well?

In the months following Tom Strong's death in August of 1972, rumors and gossip circulated among the Indians that mercury in the body of the dead man was ten times higher than the allowable level. An autopsy was performed, but details were not made public. "We don't know what danger there is," complained Bill Fobister, the band administrator at Grassy.

Council, composed of five councillors and the band chief, was determined to find out the real cause of Tom Strong's death. If mercury had killed Strong, he was the first recorded fatality of Minamata Disease in North America. The people of Grassy who persisted in eating fish from the polluted waters must know this. The whole world must know this. However, if Strong had died of a common heart attack, well, the people should know this also.

At council's direction, Fobister sent a letter to Ontario's chief coroner, H. B. Cotnam, requesting an immediate inquest to allay or confirm fears that Tom Strong died of mercury poisoning. The inquest was needed, he wrote, "so the community at Grassy Narrows could see how high mercury could be in one man who ate fish and maybe at the same time . . . learn what has been found about the different levels of mercury."

"If we must change our diet to stay healthy, we want to find out more information and especially what mercury poisoning can do to a person . . ."

"We write to you and hope you will understand why we need more information on what eating too much fish may be doing to us. We think that if everybody here could come to such an inquest and see how much mercury level is thought to be dangerous . . . this may be very important to us and our children."

Dr. Cotnam agreed to the Indians' request and called an inquest for January 1973, in Kenora. In the depths of a bleak Canadian winter, about fifty of Tom Strong's friends and family boarded a chartered bus at Grassy Narrows for the arduous ride through the bush to town.

The testimony they heard, like the rumors, was conflicting and inconclusive. The five-man inquest jury was told that the autopsy revealed Tom Strong had died from an acute coronary thrombosis, a congestion of the heart. Dr. Gordon Stopps, the government's mercury expert, said mercury levels were low and he noted that most residents at Grassy were healthy despite the mercury in their waterways.

Later, in an interview, Dr. Stopps said a precise measurement of mercury in the guide's body was impossible to obtain because there was a lapse of two or three days between his death and the autopsy. Samples taken for mercury tests were "contaminated."

At least one member of the jury, Peter Seymour, was torn by the knowledge that whatever verdict was reached would have a deep and lasting effect on the people of Grassy Narrows. Seymour, a community development officer for the Ontario government, was serving as foreman of the jury. "If we bring in a certain verdict, say of no mercury contributing to his death, these people will start eating the fish again and not be worried about its effects," Seymour explained as the jury prepared to retire. "But if we bring in a verdict that it did contribute to the death, then maybe the people will stop eating the stuff."

However, lacking anything more than a suspicion of mercury's impact on Tom Strong, the jury could only conclude that he had died of a heart attack. Pointing out the "potential danger to humans" of mercury in fish, the jury suggested that any future suspicious deaths on either of the two affected reserves should immediately become coroner's cases, subject to a thorough autopsy and inquest.

Also, the jury stated, "we recommend that the people of the English River system and the Wabigoon River area — this includes the Grassy Narrows and Whitedog Reserves — be tested annually for mercury levels during July and August (peak fishing months). There should also be regular testing for mercury content in fish in the . . . river system and the results made clearly known to the residents."

The Kenora newspaper, the *Daily Miner and News*, strangely perceived the inquest as an exercise that could not help but "calm the fears of those who have eaten considerable fish taken from the waters of the Wabigoon and English rivers."

"For, despite the fact that the deceased ate pickerel for an extended period of time, the level of mercury in his body was not excessive. According to expert testimony, the level of mercury in his system was not a contributory cause of death."

Kenora residents, especially those who owned small businesses, were anxious to be convinced that mercury had not killed Tom Strong. The town was hurting. American exchange through the local banks was off by about $5 million, and that was hard to take in a town of 10,000 persons whose economy depended heavily on tourism.

The townspeople blamed the media for printing and broadcasting inaccurate, sloppy generalizations which left the impression that all of northwestern Ontario was a polluted wasteland. Although only ten lakes along the Wabigoon and English chain were affected, in the mind of the misinformed potential visitor, the entire district, with its thousands of rivers and lakes, was contaminated.

Town residents were aware of the irony in the fact that Dryden was continuing to boom as Kenora smarted from the effects of its industry's polluting practices. But they found it hard to laugh. Further embarrassment was caused by an eighteen-foot-high replica of a muskellunge, erected in 1967 on the town's outskirts as a pollution-prevention symbol: "Husky the Muskie says Prevent Water Pollution."

Like most small towns, Kenora harbored a deep sense of municipal pride, rooted in its historic past as an early trading terminus and its present beauty as a tourist mecca. At its doorstep was the inviting unpolluted Lake of the Woods, and in its backyard were 3,000 square miles of north country within reach by road, rail, plane and boat.

But the town also experienced tensions uncommon in other communities. Kenora was situated near the Manitoba border, a thousand miles from the Ontario capital of Toronto, and its citizens felt alienated from the powerful south by distance and temperament. They naturally felt greater identi-fication with Winnipeg, a three-hour drive west, than with Toronto, a day or more away. And there were other facts of northern life that caused divisiveness.

Several Indian reserves were within driving distance of town and increasing numbers of native people came to Kenora to shop as well as for amusement. Kenorans, who were offended by the Indians' public displays, especially when intoxicated, grew openly hostile to the Indians. Some shops and restaurants barred Indians, drunk or sober, until four hundred natives from across the district marched on the town in 1965 and demanded that the town council smash the color bar and correct other discriminatory practices. Conditions improved, but esteem for the Indians did not increase. At best, the Indian presence was tolerated. At worst, it was resented to the point there was violence and open hatred on the part of both groups.

The crash of the tourist industry accentuated the tension between the two races. Idled fishermen and guides from Grassy and Whitedog increased the number of native people looking for something to do in Kenora; some were looking for trouble. They arrived in monthly waves, with their welfare cheques, willingly paying the $45 taxi fare for the one-way trip in from the reserve, or sharing the cost of a jalopy, which could be readily junked along the Jones Road if it failed to make the trip. Usually by autumn, dozens of wrecks spotted the roadside bush.

The resentment they carried with them into town frequently was fueled by cheap wines, bought by the bottle in the Liquor Control Board of

Ontario store on Kenora's main street. Drunkenness was escape, and escape was relief from the brutal realities of being Indian in a hostile time.

"I don't blame them for getting drunk sometimes," said Kenora Mayor James (Jim) Davidson. "They meet somebody and they can't resist. He's got a bottle and when they've had a few their resistance is further lowered and if someone else can afford a bottle, well they have a good time, or they forget their suffering."

"I wonder how they feel? This white man, who stained his skin and lived as a black man a few years ago. It was pretty terrible. He could feel the oppression and the lack of sympathy. 'Don't step out of line, black man.' Well, I wonder if the Indians feel that? I'd be apt to take a drink too if I had to live like that."

Many Kenorans hoped that the inquest verdict on Tom Strong's death would dampen the mercury scare and its effects on the town. But the people of Grassy Narrows returned home unconvinced. They were sure the crisis was being manipulated by the white man at their expense. That month, two stillbirths were recorded at Whitedog.

In the weeks following the Strong inquest, there was a flurry of activity at Queen's Park. William Davis had taken a tough stance on environmental issues when he led the Progressive Conservatives to a landslide victory fifteen months earlier, in the fall of 1971. Now, his administration had to demonstrate its words were not hollow. In early March of 1973, a task force was sent to Grassy and Whitedog to confer with the Indians.

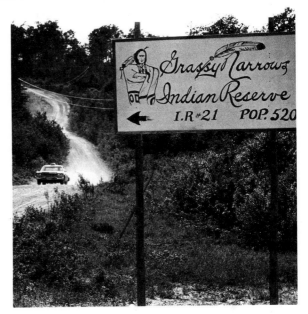

Taxi to Kenora.

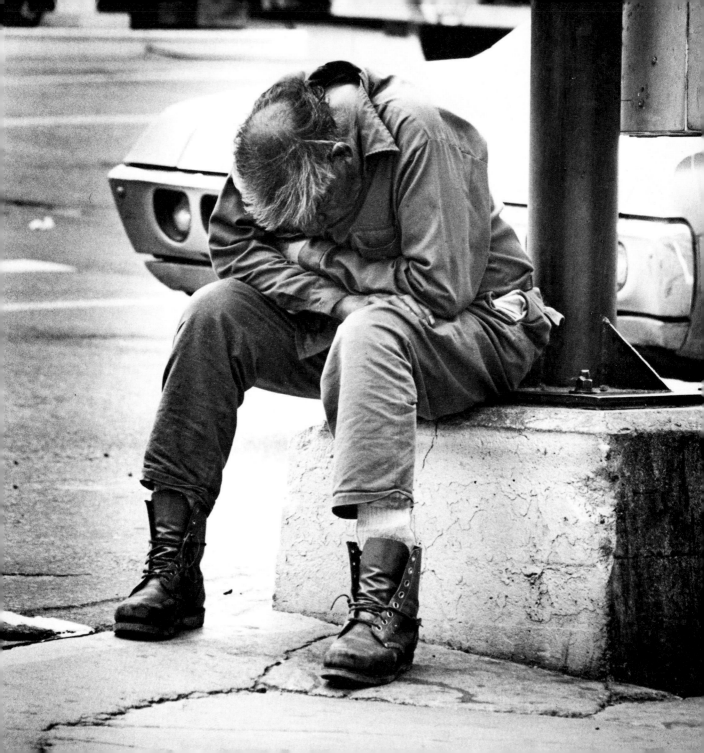

Andy Keewatin greeted the government representatives and escorted them to the community hall. Most of the Indians had come and the hall was crowded. The band council presented a brief appealing for help, to enable Grassy to deal with its social and medical problems. Council asked that a committee of Indians and government representatives be established to work on a program of recovery.

"Our people have been relocated within the past decade and we are still suffering the effects of this social upheaval," the council told the task force. "Our housing is extremely inadequate; there have been ten house fires in the past year and on the average they have burnt to the ground within a half hour. The dislocation in our lives has resulted in an excessive number of tragic deaths, violence, alcohol abuse, broken families, school drop-outs.

"All these are symptoms of our way of life now which is very much disrupted. In addition to the above situations, we also lost our commercial fishing and nearby guiding livelihoods owing to the mercury pollution. We have undergone many tests on the effects of mercury on our health and we are still in the dark as to what to do about the mercury problem."

The council said it wanted help from "top-notch resource people" — medical authorities, social workers, dieticians, lawyers, economists and community planners.

"It is experts that we need," the council said, "not local civil servants. We ask all these things not

Kenora street scene (left).

only for ourselves but for our children and for all the unborn children who must find a meaningful way in our community both present and future. We especially urge a constant surveillance of our next generations to discover the effects of mercury contamination on young children."

The council explained that only through expert study of all options open to the reserve would it be possible to "come to terms realistically with our economic, social and legal problems which have resulted from our dislocation and the mercury pollution . . ."

A spokesman for the task force said he would relay the requests to the government, but could make no promises. The task force included representatives of six provincial ministries. (The ministries were formed in a reorganization of government. Some departments were amalgamated into new groupings. One which emerged was a ministry of the environment, headed by George Kerr.)

One of the government men thanked the Indians for attending and said how much he sympathized with the hardship being experienced by families at Grassy. Tests on some band members had been completed and the mercury levels discovered were sufficiently high to make him repeat that fish consumption should be reduced. Pregnant women, or women who might become pregnant, should eat no fish at all. He explained that mercury could harm unborn children.

The audience stirred in embarrassment when the official asked if there were any questions. There was an uncomfortable pause, then a man asked: "Now that you've made us sick, what do you have to make us well?"

Dr. Gordon Stopps, the Ontario health ministry's expert on environmental health, was momentarily nonplused, but gave the only reply he could. Nothing, he said. Mercury damage to the human body was irreversible.

The meeting was short. The officials fielded questions about degrees of risk and the lack of alternate food sources and assured the people their concerns would be expressed to the authorities at Queen's Park. The women had prepared refreshments, but the government men did not stay.

Dr. Stopps distributed envelopes to some of the band members and the officials left. Nervous laughter filled the room as the Indians read out their mercury readings — 45 parts per billion — 96 ppb — 38 ppb — 289 ppb.

Matthew Beaver blushed with the embarrassment of having recorded the highest level. Some victims in Minamata, Japan, had absorbed similar amounts, although fatal doses often ran as high as 1000 ppb in blood. A resident in an uncontaminated city might expect a blood level no higher than 20 ppb. Matthew laughed nervously in response to all the teasing he was getting from his friends, but he was scared.

Marion Lamm, who had been invited by the band to attend the meeting, suggested Matthew try an easy test. "Can you touch your nose, like this?" she asked. Marion extended an arm, bringing the index finger around in a broad sweep to the tip of her nose. As Matthew tried it, the group formed a circle around him. The handsome young Indian was

the center of attention, the star of the sad show. But he touched his nose.

"Can you stand on one leg?" Marion Lamm asked.

He failed. He lifted his left leg, but his right leg wobbled and he dropped his foot to regain his balance. He tried raising his right leg, and failed once again.

Others lifted their legs and stood like flamingos, without swaying. "Look," they boasted. "It's easy. Like this." But the more he tried, the more unsteady he became, and the fright he felt in his gut showed in his face.

They don't understand, thought Marion. They just don't understand. That had been a test for Minamata Disease.

Matthew Beaver had been having problems with his balance for some time, but like other men on the reserve he had been drinking a lot lately. Still, his fear increased as he thought about the trouble he had been having lately with his eyes.

"I can see if I look straight ahead," he said, "but if my cap is on the seat beside me, I can't see it."

On its return to Toronto, the task force made a quick and concise report to Natural Resources Minister Leo Bernier, recommending that immediate steps be taken to help the reserves and rid the uncontaminated regions of the stigma of mercury pollution.

"It was evident," the task force reported, "that the Indian problems were complicated and that these were not just the result of mercury pollution, but the latter had created quite a disruption of their way of life, their employment habits and their livelihood; that some action was required to assist the Indians to replace the position guiding and commercial fishing had in their way of life before the two bands could hope to have anything approaching a stable community life."

The task force recommended that alternative food supplies be provided to the Indians, financial assistance as compensation and loans be provided both Indians and camp operators, and a prohibition placed on the taking of fish for food from the affected waters, "recognizing that complete closure of the waters to all forms of fishing may have to take place for control purposes."

The task force was sufficiently concerned about the Indians' health to recommend "examinations of the population most at risk be carried out in greater depth at the earliest possible moment."

"Welfare is in danger of becoming an accepted way of life among the Indian people and there are few meaningful occupations available to them," the advisors told Bernier. "Frequent use of alcohol, drugs and other sought-after stimuli in conjunction with periodic outbreaks of crime and violence have combined to produce inflated welfare costs and a deterioration in the social life of the band communities."

"Although the detrimental effect of the mercury problem is by no means the sole contributing factor to the deteriorating social conditions, it would appear to have played a significant role, although not readily definable."

The task force concluded the federal government was responsible in large measure for the conditions beyond those directly related to mercury pollution and proposed close co-operation between the senior governments to clean up the mess.

It was critically blunt about the health threat, which had been ignored for nearly three years. "Fish from the Wabigoon and Lower English River system," the task force told Bernier, "[should] not be used for human or animal food."

Bernier promised to establish a long-range program for socio-economic redevelopment, an alternate food supply of fish from unpolluted waters and jobs in an expanded forest industry, a bittersweet proposal. But he was not prepared to shut down the river system, again fearing the enormous consequences in terms of compensation.

Instead, then Health Minister Richard Potter announced that he was distributing pamphlets alerting northern residents to the dangers of eating the contaminated fish. The action angered Liberal critic Patrick Reid of Rainy River, who pointed out, "They can't eat those damn booklets."

About the time Bernier was making his promises of corrective measures, the Canadian Civil Liberties Education Trust was coincidentally completing a study of the Indian and Canadian law.

"Ever since white man's arrival in North America," the trust noted, "he has increasingly encroached upon the Indian's domain. An expanding white society has usurped Indian hunting ground, polluted Indian waters, invaded Indian trap lines and commandeered Indian land. . . .

"Too often, senior levels of government content

themselves with the statutory enshrinement of empty slogans. Once having secured the enactment of a promising statute, our governments virtually retreat from the problem. They don't ask enough questions, plug enough loopholes or vote enough money. The follow-through in the community rarely matches the rhetoric in the Legislature.

"Regrettably, for all their promises and pronouncements, Canadian lawmakers are doing far too little to amend the deterioration."

As the experience of three years had shown, politicians seemed to be incapable of coming to grips with the mercury crisis. Part of the failure could be traced to a general lack of co-ordination between federal and provincial authorities. In proposing closer co-operation between the senior levels of government, the task force on mercury was calling for a drastic departure from past political practice.

The federal government in Ottawa was Liberal. The provincial government in Toronto was Conservative. The responsibility for Indian affairs was federal. The responsibility for pollution control was provincial. But the crisis would not fit between neat jurisdictional lines. It overlapped, affecting other complex federal-provincial jurisdictions where costs and responsibilities were shared — health, welfare, education, labor.

Political realities made it possible for the Liberals in Ottawa to place the responsibility for solutions on the shoulders of Ontario's Tories, and vice versa. When political considerations prevailed, the Indians were bound to suffer.

Bernier's plan to help the Indians was well-meaning, if half-hearted. He proposed pilot projects to expand employment opportunities and a food program to replace lost protein. First, standard freezers, then larger, walk-in units would be installed on the reserves and men hired to fish nearby unpolluted waters. The program was destined to fail. The people preferred fresh fish to frozen fish, and if American sportsmen could continue to fish the English River, why, the Indians asked, couldn't they? The frozen fish accumulated, they were eaten only when fishing on the polluted waters just off their shores was unproductive.

As minister of natural resources, Bernier was anxious to stimulate the exploitation of the north's abundant store of minerals and timber. But pressure from environmentalists forced him to tread cautiously. As a good politician, Bernier knew what to do; in March 1973, he appointed a committee which would advise on all matters affecting the ministry.

Again, he stumbled into a hornet's nest of criticism and controversy. One of his first choices for membership on the committee was T. S. (Tom) Jones, the vice-president of Anglo-Canadian Pulp and Paper, and manager of the Dryden mill.

"This appointment is totally inept and inappropriate," protested Stephen Lewis, the recently chosen leader of the New Democratic party.

"It ties the whole industry in with the ministry [of natural resources]," Lewis said. "He turns to the industry for his advisory committee, a firm involved in the . . . pollution of the northwest."

Jones' views on northern development were well known. He spoke out against ill-founded southern pronouncements "from people who really are lacking in their knowledge of the north" and stressed that there was plenty of room for the logger and the vacationer.

"It is possible to have wilderness areas, and we have some, and we possibly need more," he said. "But other legitimate users should not be denied access to the forests and their use without every consideration being given to wise use by and for the people."

He contended that to achieve this wise use, the pulp and paper industry needed help from government in overcoming rising costs, high federal taxation, increased freight rates and a depressed market.

"In no way are we asking as an industry for special consideration," he said. "We will pay our fair tax share quite willingly. But the present tax burden only makes the Canadian industry non-competitive in the world market. The outlook without government action is not encouraging."

Government was not unsympathetic to the industry's plea for consideration. The provincial government, for example, had been giving Anglo-Canadian tax rebates on equipment under its pollution-control incentive program – $18,957.35. In fact, Queen's Park was giving $821,113.53 to Dow Chemical, the company it was suing for $25 million.

If Jones' comments could be taken at face value, he would clearly be expected to advise Bernier to expand the existing timber-cutting limits while dealing sympathetically with the over-taxed

industry. Considering Bernier's avowed desire for northern development and increased jobs, he could be expected to comply.

As spring returned to English River country in 1973, the camps re-opened, their operators by now thoroughly committed to downplaying the mercury problem in their waters. Government loans only added to the financial burdens they must shoulder. Survival was vital, and the operators did what they could to survive.

"We feel the rumors regarding the so-called mercury pollution have been highly overrated, and reports have been blown way out of proportion, to be highly misleading," the operator of Grassy Lodge, not far from the reserve, wrote one guest.

"We have continued to eat fish from our waters, on a regular basis, without ill effect. We have a letter from the minister of the Ontario department of lands and forests, which states 'Tests have been run on natives of northwestern Ontario whose diets contained a large portion of fish, with a high mercury content. Even in these people, no clinical symptoms of mercury poisoning were found. Nowhere in Ontario have any cases of mercury poisoning been found. Nowhere in Ontario have any cases of mercury poisoning occurred.'

" . . . The unspoiled beauties of nature on our many lakes, combined with the fabulous fishing, makes your stay at Grassy Lodge a restful one, which will long be remembered."

Even the anglers, by now, had rationalized their presence on the mercury-polluted waters. "I think it's always been there," said a vacationing farmer

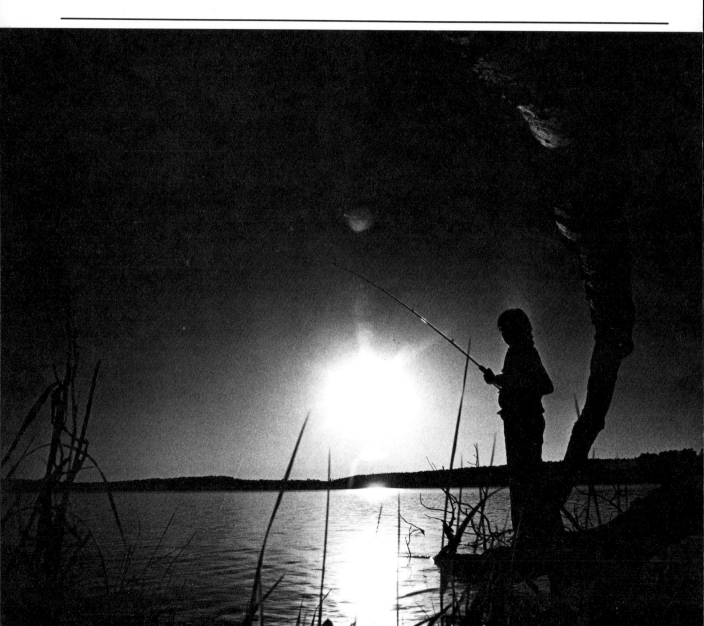

from Michigan. "They've just found a way of reading it. It's like the feed we were giving our cattle. They found mercury in it, so we can't use that feed no more." He turned to a fishing friend. "How much did they say you had to eat before you'd get mercury poisoning, Jim?"

"Somethin' like two pounds a day for twenty years," his buddy replied.

"Yeah. Two pounds a day for twenty years, Nobody eats that much."

Back in Kenora, Barney and Marion Lamm were packing their belongings. Barney was expanding his air service in a hangar alongside an abandoned wartime training strip in Gimli, Manitoba. They had decided to make their home there. The atmosphere in Kenora had grown too hostile.

"The talk around town and the attitude of the people is that it is our fault," Marion complained. "It isn't the mercury. It isn't the fact that the government announced it. It is our fault. We have stuck it out for three summers, but that's enough."

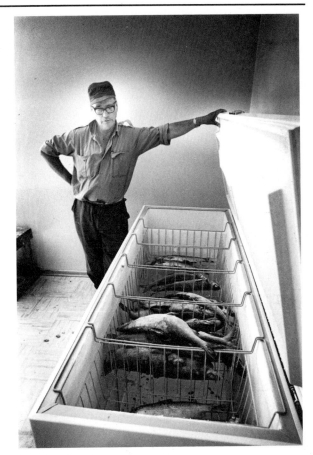

Andy Keewatin with government freezer, 1975.

7

It's a Good Day to Die, White Man

Just looking at the population, you can't say that mercury has done this to the people, because it's such a vague kind of thing. But they have the blood levels which, it has been shown, have these effects in industrial populations. It has probably had a direct medical impact on the reserve, but a much more profound effect is the interference with the economy — the disintegration of the family, the alcoholism . . . it's horrendous.

—Dr. Peter Newberry
Grassy Narrows, 1975

The children of Grassy Narrows suffered as much as their troubled parents. Alcohol was ostensibly prohibited on the reserve by treaty, and whenever the adults left in search of beer and wine, which was often, the youngsters would pursue their own route of escape.

Most were unable to afford or obtain beer or liquor, but there were other ways to bend the mind and forget the present; less palatable ways, but effective. Gas was siphoned from abandoned jalopies, parked cars or outboard motors. Magic Markers were stolen from the school, broken open and sniffed. There was a run on nail polish remover and shaving lotion at the Hudson's Bay store.

Teachers noticed that two or three of the suspected "chronic" gas sniffers were developing difficulties with their studies, and the truancy rate increased. Some children arrived for class nursing hangovers, or even drunk from a morning date with a gas can.

Weekends were particularly bad. The reserve was almost deserted by adults who took cabs or hitched rides into Kenora. Left to fend for them-

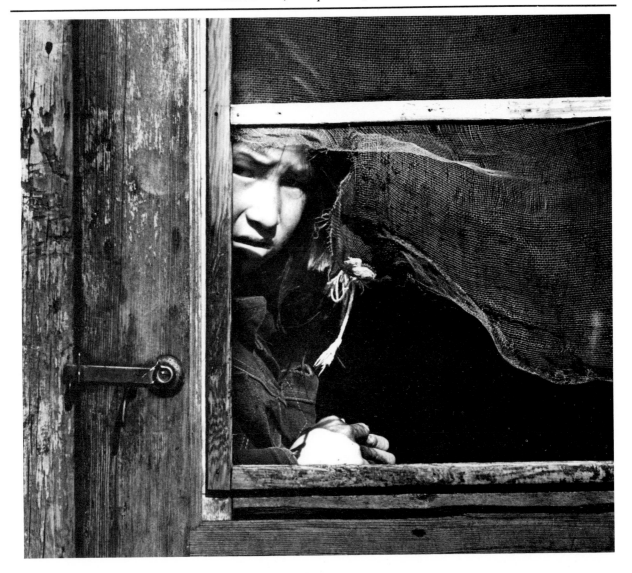

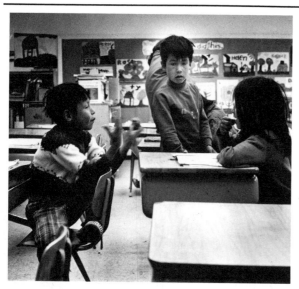

Grassy Narrows school.

selves, the children roamed the reserve in packs, long into the night, satisfying their mischievous whims at will. Ironically, the damage they caused had to be repaired, and so provided partial employment for jobless men.

On the return of the adults to the reserve, the children were often terrorized, subjected to beatings or compelled to watch one drunken parent attack the other. Many sought refuge at the lodge of a group of Mennonites, on the edge of the reserve.

A researcher reported to the federal department of health and welfare that "because the older people drink, the young people also indulge, and because there [are] no laws governing the drinking of hard beverages on the reserve, save for the one that states 'Liquor shall not be taken to the reserve,' when liquor did start coming in illegally, as it is doing now, there was no rule or order as to its consumption."

"It seems that the people who drink, drink to excess," commented Dennis Clark, principal of the Grassy Narrows School. "Not that everyone who drinks is an alcoholic. But they don't do social drinking the way we define it. Their social drinking is a weekend blast. Maybe there is a reason for them to get drunk."

"The drinking pattern is that they will drink until there is nothing left, or they can't drink any-more and pass out. Then, the kids get into the remaining beer or whiskey and they drink the same way they see their parents drink. Since the children don't have the same access to alcohol as the parents do, they also go gas sniffing. Not just gas sniffing. The kids go to solvents."

Sandlot hockey.

The Bay store.

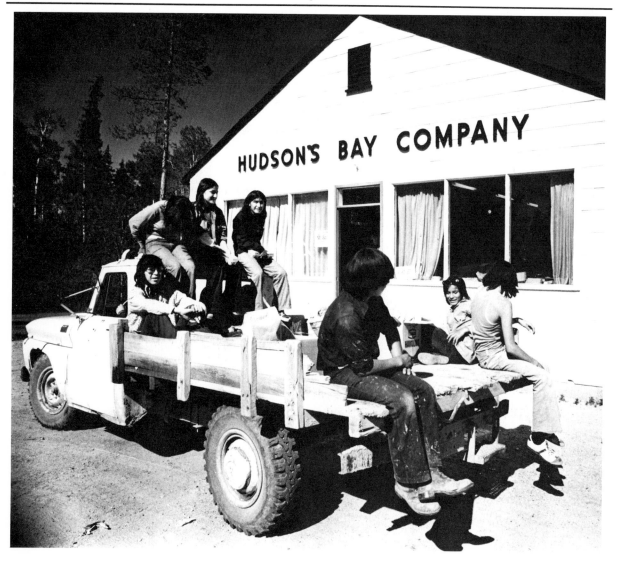

Physician William Parker of the Deer Lodge Hospital in Winnipeg said Grassy Narrows, like other reserves, should concern itself less about mercury and more about solving the problem of alcohol and gas sniffing. He found no evidence of mercury poisoning in autopsies performed on some residents of Grassy, but said brain damage could be anticipated, especially among young people, from lead additives in gasoline.

"In this province [Manitoba] we have a terribly high incidence of gasoline sniffing," he said. "The gasoline they have been using has been lead-additive gas and the lead compound, with the anti-knocking agent in the gasoline, is volatile. We have evidence here of chronic lead-intoxication."

"I would suggest that they spend more time looking for lead in Ontario than mercury," he said, "because I think it is a much more widespread and definite problem that I can put my finger on."

"Gas is the only thing the kids can get. When the mother and father go on a binge with alcohol, the kids have a party with gasoline. It's the only thing they can get up there, from outboards and tractors and so on."

With the spring of 1974, four full years after the discovery of mercury in the waters of English River country, violence and alcohol-related deaths had been woven into the pattern of life at Grassy Narrows. The tragedy of Grassy had reached such proportions that solutions which might have been considered workable when the pollution was first discovered were by now increasingly less practical. The federal and provincial governments fell back on traditional methods of keeping dependent native peoples busy — homebuilding, construction of recreation facilities, logging and general make-work projects.

Grander plans were in the works for northwestern Ontario generally. In 1971, the provincial government had received and endorsed a task force report entitled "Design for Development", which proposed that the pulp and paper industry be encouraged to make better use of the northern forests. The report suggested between four thousand and five thousand new jobs could be created by increasing the harvest in a balanced forestry program.

Bernier invited the pulp and paper industry to submit plans for expansion into the area. Some companies disclosed programs to increase cuts in existing timber limits, but Anglo-Canadian expressed a desire to expand its Dryden plant and perhaps build a new mill in the area of Ear Falls, or Red Lake, far to the north of Grassy Narrows.

In the Ontario Legislature on March 7, 1974, Premier William Davis announced the government's endorsement of the company's plans. He said if preliminary studies were confirmed, the Dryden operation would grow and a new kraft pulp mill, sawmill, fiberboard plant and specialty chemical plant would be constructed.

"If all projects prove feasible and are proceeded with," said Davis, "there would be a total investment of $253 million resulting in approximately 1800 new jobs by 1978 in the pulp mills, in the sawmills and in the woodlands. This would be double

Last fall, we launched a tree-planting program in Grassy Narrows.
Leo Bernier

the number of people the company now employs in northwestern Ontario."

The premier said the development program was consistent with the government's "Design for Development" of the northwest. What the premier did not disclose was that the company's plans would eventually require timber rights over a vast tract of virgin forest — almost nineteen thousand square miles along the fifty-first parallel, a region as large as the province of Nova Scotia.

The desired territory was carpeted with black spruce, a slow-growing tree which had escaped the chain saw and cutting rigs until now because of its relative inaccessibility along Canada's tree line. Up here, trees and people continued to survive in a most delicate balance with nature. As many as two thousand Cree and Ojibway Indians lived within the tract. Another three thousand lived near trap lines which extended into the area.

Davis implied there was no reason to worry about the company's grandiose scheme. "Close co-operation between Anglo-Canadian and the Ontario government will be maintained to ensure that all necessary efforts are made to protect the environment." He said the company was planning to spend $2.5 million to build a new chlor-alkali plant at Dryden "using new non-mercury technology" to eliminate the final traces of the element from the company's operations.

Stephen Lewis, the New Democratic party leader, had not forgotten the appointment a year earlier of T. S. Jones, vice-president of Anglo-Canadian, to an advisory committee in Leo Bernier's ministry of natural resources.

"As I recall," said Lewis, "he is one of the chief executive officers. Is he also a senior adviser, perhaps chairman of the advisory committee to the minister of natural resources?"

"No," Bernier curtly replied.

"He is not an adviser to the minister of natural resources?" Lewis persisted.

"He stepped down last November," Bernier said.

"He stepped down in November?" Lewis quizzically repeated, then shook his head. "That answers my question."

There was no reason to assume that Indians would benefit from jobs in the expanding pulp and paper industry. Bernier readily admitted that the skills of the unemployed men at Grassy Narrows and Whitedog were not suited to this kind of work.

"Last fall, we launched a tree-planting program in Grassy Narrows and couldn't find enough Indians to fill the requirements," he said. The ministry also gave Grassy a cutting area from which five thousand cords of wood could have been cut. Whitedog was allowed a three thousand cord maximum. Only three hundred cords were harvested by each band.

"Well," Bernier remarked, "I have to admit that pulp cutting is tough work. The problem is, how do you give one of these people, say in their forties, who are used to the traditional ways of trapping and fishing, a power saw and say 'Okay, cut down those trees?' It's not easy for them."

"Our people are working with them, trying to motivate them," Bernier said. "It will take time.

What has really caught the Indians in a bind is inflation.
Leo Bernier

We freed up more areas for trap lines and even helped in relocating these lines, but the response was not encouraging."

He said the Indians were also given access to uncontaminated lakes, four or five miles from the reserves, but few would bother to travel the distance to fish the lakes. "Only the ones that are ambitious do it."

But, Bernier concluded, there is "no real suffering. About 90 per cent of the reserves get government assistance of one kind or another. What has really caught the Indians in a bind is inflation. For example, the cost of sugar has gone away up, and they think it is only happening in their particular area."

Bernier was underestimating the seriousness of the problems faced by the native people; he was also oversimplifying the answers to those problems. However, the prices being charged at the nearby Hudson's Bay store were a matter of legitimate concern. The National Indian Brotherhood, in the course of its investigations into the impact of mercury pollution, discovered that at the Bay commodities such as eggs, hamburger, apples and soda pop could carry a price tag twice as high as that of similar items on sale in Kenora. Ten pounds of sugar sold for as much as $14.70, five dollars higher than in town.

The Indian brotherhood used the results of its survey to appeal to the provincial government for a flight plan which would enable Indian fishermen to fly north into unpolluted lakes as an interim measure to replace lost protein. "Fish as a protein source — caught by the native people themselves — is urgently needed on the reserves," the brotherhood stated. "Many people cannot afford to eat the expensive food for sale at Grassy." The government rejected the airlift proposal.

The government had money to spend on projects, but its investments tended to be more visible elsewhere, such as the bankroll being sunk into Minaki Lodge, the aging resort on the Winnipeg River chain, about thirty miles west of Grassy Narrows.

Minaki was a handsome place, built by the Canadian National Railway in 1927 on a rolling hundred-acre site overlooking the route of the early voyageurs and fur traders. The grounds included a golf course and cabins. The mercury scare had severely damaged business and Barney Lamm had divested himself of his 10 per cent share. By 1974, the government had lent its private owners about $1.1 million and finally took over its operation with plans to transform it into a 200-room year-round recreation and convention facility.

Tourism Minister Claude Bennett said Minaki's financial affairs would be put in order and the government was working on the scheme "to make Minaki Lodge a jewel in the necklace of tourist facilities that threads throughout Ontario."

Bennett lacked neither words nor money. The government agreed to spend up to five million dollars on the project and Bennett said the area would have world-wide appeal for people "who will be charmed by the peace and quiet and the sheer beauty of the rivers and lakes and forests of this

Minaki Lodge, 1976.

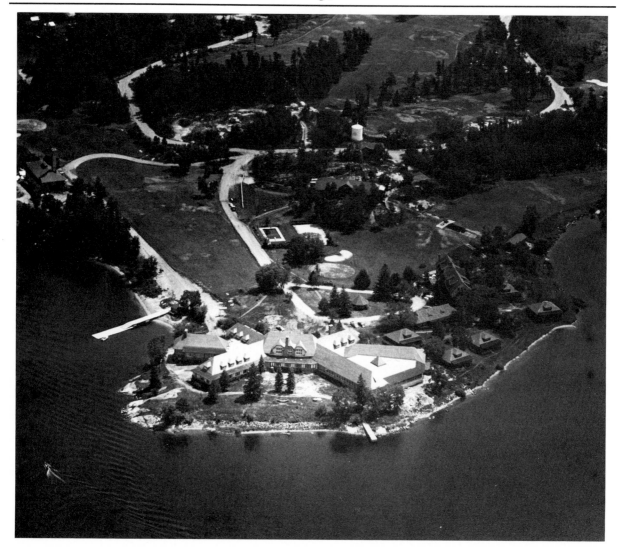

region and will visit again and again.... We propose to seize the future."

The tourism minister neglected in his enthusiasm to mention that the lodge was situated on a polluted waterway. Fish in the vicinity of the lodge had mercury levels averaging between one and two parts per million — two to four times higher than the acceptable federal standard.

Rather than emerging as a "jewel" in a necklace, the lodge rapidly became an anvil around the government's neck. Previously undetected structural defects sent costs soaring. The kitchen flooring was weak and condemned. Insulation was flammable and had to be replaced. The indoor swimming pool was sub-standard and raw sewage was found in the outdoor pool. The lodge was closed to make repairs, never to open again. The five million dollars was spent simply to bring it up to health and safety standards. Further expenditures were approved.

In January 1977, the Ontario Legislature's public accounts committee was told the government had sunk about $7.5 million into acquisition and renovation and was spending $50,000 a year to heat and guard the vacant lodge. Deficits could push total costs beyond nine million dollars, including $370,500 spent on consultants, who advised the government it would cost fifteen to eighteen million dollars to complete the original plan.

Fred Boyer, executive director of the tourism division of the Ontario ministry of industry and tourism, said it would have been cheaper to build a new resort than renovate the old lodge. And a new resort would have been constructed closer to a major traffic artery. "We wouldn't locate at Minaki," he told the legislative committee. "It's a little too difficult to get to."

Bennett appeared before the public accounts committee in February 1977, to explain the debacle and, incredibly, suggested that another $8 million might make the lodge a viable operation. He explained the original plan was based on "my own intuition, several reports and the best advice of my staff." "There was no doubt I was flying by the seat of my pants," he said. "I'm not denying that ... [but] I think the day will come when Minaki will be a viable operation in northwestern Ontario. I hope some day I'll be able to smile."

The abortive experiment at Minaki would eventually cost Ontario taxpayers twice or perhaps even triple the total amount of money spent by both the provincial and federal governments on programs at Grassy Narrows and Whitedog. So much for priorities.

Although they had moved out of the Kenora district, the Lamms kept an eye on the mercury situation in the area. Especially Marion. By now, she had accumulated a storehouse of material on the problem, including government correspondence, scientific papers, newspaper reports and magazine articles from three continents.

The articles included a story about award-winning New York photojournalist W. Eugene Smith, formerly with *Life* magazine, who was working with his Japanese-American wife Aileen on a book about the people of Minamata, a dramatic chronicle of the dreadful Japanese experience. In

**Their jobs were a source of pride,
but now they're gone.
It is a vicious circle,
because one problem breeds another.**

December 1973, Marion Lamm wrote to the Smiths inquiring if they were aware of the mercury problem in northwestern Ontario and the many similarities to Minamata. The letter raised the specter of a third outbreak of Minamata Disease.

While covering a demonstration of Minamata Disease patients against the Chisso Corporation, Smith suffered serious head injuries when knocked to the ground by company guards. He returned to the United States for treatment and in July 1974, Aileen Smith, an energetic and committed environmentalist, seized the opportunity to visit Grassy Narrows and Whitedog to gather material for a separate chapter on Canada and the Indians. The first tenuous link between the Indians and the Minamatans had been established.

The summer of 1974 was no better than the previous ones. It was the fifth summer that the Indians were being asked to spend in idleness, surrounded by an abundance of fish which they were not supposed to eat. With sportsmen plying the waters off their shores, many could not reasonably resist the temptation to fish. Meanwhile, tensions in Grassy grew. So did violence.

The people were restless, anxious to experiment with possible solutions. They decided to replace their conservative chief, Andy Keewatin, with a younger leader. They chose Tom Keesick, a twenty-five-year-old Ojibway radical who had none of Keewatin's patience.

Keesick prided himself on his knowledge of white society. He was born and raised in the railway junctions of the north, and as a rebellious youth had been confined in training school for juvenile delinquency. For a time he lived in Toronto at Rochdale College, a free school experiment which was a magnet for transient, disenchanted young people and radical thinkers. Back in the north, Keesick allied himself with Louis Cameron of Whitedog and others to form the Ojibway Warriors Society, a militant group in search of equality for Indians in central Canada.

The Ojibway Warriors Society would be heard from. Those within nearest earshot were the residents of Kenora, where whites were growing openly hostile to the continued presence of drunken Indians on the streets. Young whites were seen beating intoxicated Indians and older residents shouted insults back at taunting natives.

"I don't think it's a matter of racism or discrimination," reasoned one prominent citizen. "But if, day after day, a particular group is stretched out on the street so you have to step over them, so drunk that they can't stand up, you are going to have people crying about it."

He acknowledged that the scene was a national disgrace, reminiscent of the black-white conflicts in the southern United States. But part of the problem was the mercury pollution, with all of its economic implications.

"Their jobs were a source of pride, but now they're gone. It is a vicious circle, because one problem breeds another. I suppose you could call the white reaction racism. But it's very specifically against drunkenness, because it is prevalent." In 1973 Kenora recorded 6,900 arrests for public

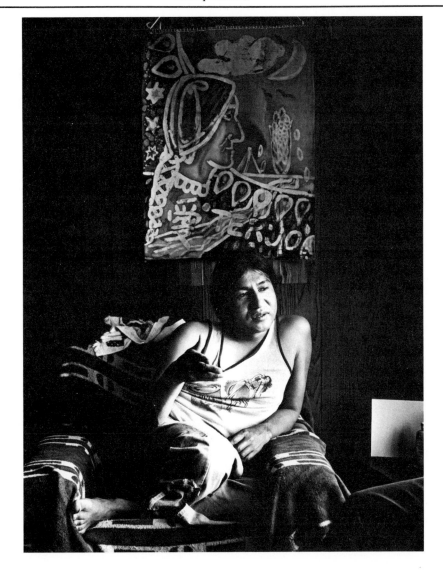

drunkenness.

"I grew up in this area, which meant growing up with a great many Indian people. I see fellas I went to school with on the street, drunk, and I know damn well they could have gone anywhere they wanted, as far as intelligence goes. But they got into a rut and fell by the wayside. Mercury has been a contributing factor. There has been a complete social upheaval."

Perhaps time had distorted his view of the past. Kenora for years had been widely known as a rugged town where Indians were given a hard time. But he preferred to remember it as a "busy, vibrant, lively community" rather than a place of drunken violence. "It's a bitter community right now," he said. "It's not the same place I grew up in."

Queen's Park was not unaware of the problem. In May 1974, Premier William Davis had sent a group of cabinet ministers to Kenora. Margaret Birch, provincial secretary for social development, headed the delegation. They saw drunks in grimy clothes staggering along Main Street, victims of hangovers sleeping in parks, outbursts among Indians who loitered on street corners, people who had nowhere to go, nothing to do. And if their eyes didn't see their ears heard.

"The human degradation that results from the abuse of alcohol alone is plainly evident on the main street of Kenora and along the waterfront," Mayor Jim Davidson said.

Researchers for the Grand Council of the Treaty Three district completed a study in 1973 which documented 189 violent deaths of native people in the Kenora area between January 1970, and June 1973 — more than one every week, 70 per cent linked to alcohol abuse.

The victims were primarily young men, women and children. Youngsters under the age of ten appeared as regular victims of violence. Several died in tent and house fires, set intentionally or by accident by their parents. Suicides were common among young people and alcohol-poisoning claimed at least a dozen lives.

The study, entitled "While People Sleep", revealed that during the 42-month period 38 persons died of gunshot wounds, stabbing or hanging, 30 in fires, 42 drowned, 25 perished from exposure and 16 died in car crashes. "We must look beyond the statistics, lest they lead us to view the problems with cold detachment," the council stated. "We must understand that what we are looking at is a tragedy to public and private agencies in many millions of dollars a year. The cost in human suffering is incalculable."

Mayor Davidson suggested that people whose futures are so unpromising stop caring about their own lives, those of their friends and their children. He cited public defecation, copulation and violence as "symptoms of a moral pollution that deserves more attention than all the efforts now being made to eliminate sources of environmental pollution."

Birch, the secretary for social development, said: "I've never seen anything like it anywhere." The cabinet members agreed that something should be done, but first a large-scale study of the whole social question, with special emphasis on Kenora, was

"It's a good day to die, white man."
"Any day is a good day to die, son."

needed. With that, Birch led her colleagues back to Toronto.

The federal government was equally cautious. The young militants of the Ojibway Warrior Society had long before stopped believing that any officer sent by the Indian Affairs department could do anything to change things for them. In July, a group of area Indians, and others from the United States and western Canada, sought and received permission from the mayor to hold a three-day conference in Anicinabe Park, a fourteen-acre treed area on the outskirts of town, regularly used for camping by Indians and tourists on travels through the district. The conference dwelt on inequities long endured by native peoples, and the continuing white invasion of traditional Indian lands.

Rhetoric stirred emotions and the conference quickly turned into a militant demonstration. Led by Louis Cameron of Whitedog, a lean man who spoke softly but tough, about 150 Indians — mostly in their teens and early twenties — decided that Anicinabe Park should be reclaimed as the rightful possession of Treaty Three Indians.

Barricades were erected at park entrances and rifles were brought in to reinforce claims. In idle moments, Molotov cocktails were manufactured with bottles and gasoline and rags, and tested against rocks. Anicinabe Park had become an occupied zone and the attention of white North Americans became fixed on Kenora and its troubles.

The air was charged but, in its early stages, the occupation had a bizarre, carnival-like appeal. Townspeople and tourists flocked to the suburban refuge, driving leisurely along the winding road that formed the park border. Indians, toting rifles, fired only obscenities. But the atmosphere rapidly turned ugly. An early spokesman for the militants was Harvey Major, a former hair stylist from Des Moines, Iowa, a middle-aged Indian who had gained press attention a year earlier when the American Indian Movement (AIM) laid siege to Wounded Knee. With typical bravado, Major warned: "If just one of our Indian people is hit by a bullet, Kenora will go up in smoke." Major's loose talk would soon reduce his credibility among his fellow demonstrators, but the early threat was taken seriously by those outside the occupied area, and seemed to underscore the potential for a violent outbreak which would be interpreted around the world as a racial battle.

Officers were sent in to reinforce the more than one hundred provincial policemen who had been airlifted into Kenora in advance of the conference. They remained a conspicuous presence in town. Regular patrols in black and white bubble-topped cruisers were made past the park, which had become the scene of a standoff.

One such patrol was confronted by a young warrior, his rifle at the ready, eyes brimming with defiance. He scowled at the officer, who in turn peered back at the youth through chrome-rimmed sunglasses "It's a good day to die, white man," the Indian taunted. The policeman lowered his glasses and said through the open window of his cruiser: "Any day is a good day to die, son."

The uneasy peace was occasionally broken. A

contractor trying to salvage building materials from a house under construction near the park took off on a dead run when shots were fired over his head. A nearby resort operator said a bullet also whizzed over his head.

Derek Hodgson, a reporter with the Toronto *Globe and Mail*, had been allowed by Indian leaders into the park to report their demands and the nature of the demonstration, but his reports from inside the park ceased abruptly after a young Indian pointed a double-barrelled shotgun at Hodgson's head and pulled the trigger. The hammer clicked. The youth loaded the gun and fired a shot at a nearby bush. Hodgson hit the youth with his camera and later referred to him as a "thug" in a report of the incident. The Indian warriors then closed the barricade to all reporters.

There were also moving moments inside the occupation zone, as the young warriors, sought to recapture their traditional heritage. They conferred with their elders and performed drum dances and gathered in small knots to weigh past values against present pressures. Under canvas and a full moon, it seemed almost possible to attain a balance between the two. But, outside the park, the police patrolled.

Indian demands were many, and involved all three levels of government, from municipal to federal. Primarily, they claimed ownership of the park on behalf of the native people, saying it had been illegally sold to the town by the white man. They also insisted, however, on the swift resolution of a score of grievances.

Among them were an investigation into the evidence of rising violent death among native peoples; more job opportunities in Kenora; an Indian patrol to assist town police in coping with Indian problems; fuller and fairer coverage of Indian issues by the local news media; removal of the provincial court judge, whose sentences they considered unduly severe; immediate negotiations with Indians affected by mercury pollution; a police college for northwestern Ontario; a native council on alcoholism; equitable distribution of federal funds to Indian reserves; dismissal of all senior federal Indian Affairs employees in the Kenora district, replacing them by officials mutually acceptable to the Indians and Ottawa; increased medical and dental services; a comprehensive economic development program; better housing and improved schooling, including elementary schools on all reserves and an Indian high school for the Kenora district.

The Indians called for Mayor Davidson to conduct negotiations. A former school teacher, he presented a stern facade. But he was very much a humanist and sympathized with the Indians' terrible plight. But other town leaders did not share his willingness to bargain with natives they felt were no better than lawless thugs.

The mayor negotiated a ten-day truce with the young militants, but his conciliatory style was not popular among some townspeople, who formed a Citizens' Area Committee. They preferred to be viewed as a pressure group rather than a vigilante organization, but members called for a variety of measures, even a citizens' march on the park to take repossession. John Reid, a federal Liberal and member of Parliament for the Kenora-Rainy River riding, cautioned the group against such an action.

"When we talk of going in and cleaning them out, we are talking of bloodshed," he warned during a visit to the town.

The emergence of the citizens' committee demonstrated the polarization between the two races in Kenora, and this deep-seated mistrust eventually thwarted Davidson's efforts to talk the warriors out of Anicinabe Park. Responsibility for the negotiations shifted to Queen's Park. The Ontario government sent in a negotiator from the attorney-general's office. The occupation would be ended by consultation if possible, by force if necessary. A hundred provincial policemen stood by. The talks dragged on for weeks.

At one point, a group of Toronto Quakers (the religious Society of Friends) entered the park to talk to the warriors as part of a cross-Canada study on "justice and the Canadian Indian." They emerged with a plea for tolerance and action on the Indians' demands.

"We are convinced by our study, and especially by our Kenora visit, that the long-standing grievances and sufferings of the native people, amounting in effect to genocide, must be recognized and responded to now at last, with speedy positive action and not with attempted containment by force."

The Quakers saw the occupation as "a sign, not an end in itself."

"It will be a tragedy of great magnitude if it continues to be treated as a local legality, or if a backlash against the Indian people is allowed to develop around it.

"We believe that protests against arms-bearing and threat of violence are hypocritical in the white society. These young people protest that they bear arms because they have watched their people die in Kenora and other areas of Canada in violent and often mysterious ways, to which the law makes little or no response, and they believe all reasonable ways to justice for them have failed.

"If the governments of Canada at their various levels do not respond to the ills of their people they need not be surprised if those people refuse to acknowledge them and attempt to establish a government of their own. The young people in Anicinabe Park have a deep sense that they too are children of God and, as such, are entitled to a just and honest hearing of their grievances in this their own homeland, from the people who are elected to govern them . . . .

"We are not to complain that outside supporters, especially from the United States, are coming to the aid of their native brothers and sisters. The Indian world is united in a spiritual way and the forty-ninth parallel [the Canada-U.S. border] has no meaning for them . . . .

"We appeal to all levels of government in Canada, to the Christian churches and spiritual communities of this land, to all educational and socially concerned agencies and to all people of good will to respond to the pleas of the native people for human consideration and for justice, and to do so with imagination, trust and utmost urgency."

The negotiations with the tiny army of militants in the park were arduous and often stormy. But, finally, as the weeks wore on, agreement was reached to pursue many of the Indians' complaints and search the title to the park. The occupation ended on August 18. Twenty-seven persons, including Tommy Keesick, the activist chief from Grassy Narrows, were charged with acts of conspiracy and bearing dangerous weapons. The charges would eventually be dropped and ownership of the park once again claimed by the town.

Mayor Davidson said Kenora acted with great restraint in the face of the Indians' provocation. He said that by refusing to be drawn into a confrontation Kenora had "won the war." Davidson, however, had lost considerable public support and would be defeated for re-election by four votes as the town looked for tougher leadership. The choice was local businessman William Tomashowski, a hard-liner during the occupation.

Davidson was hurt by the defeat, but said, "If I had to do it over again I'd do it the same way." "I have sympathy for the Indians' situation," he explained. "I have no sympathy for the redneck attitude of some people who laugh at them. We have to consult them. We can't impose solutions on them. If you want someone to support something you consult them. You bring them into the decision-making process. Don't treat them like children.

"If we were subjected to the same conditions, I think we'd be raising more hell than the Indians. Yes, I have no sympathy for those who call them savages. They are not scalping savages. They are just ordinary [people] who haven't had an education, don't know too much, who live the way their parents lived, in harmony with their environment. That's not the way we live. We destroy it for the next generation. Part of their way of life would do us a lot of good."

Davidson said he felt the park occupation had served to concentrate attention on the problems confronting both the town and the native peoples.

"Until the people know there are Third World conditions at our own back door, depressed conditions, that citizens of this country are living in a certain amount of misery, a stone age existence, if they don't know it nothing will be done. So in that sense, I think the publicity did some good."

Later, Indians of the district would invite Davidson to a pow wow and award him a feathered peace pipe. "I don't know whether they are chicken feathers or eagle feathers," he said. "I'd like to think they are eagle feathers. I will treasure it very highly as a memento of my term as mayor."

Back at Grassy Narrows, the reception for Tommy Keesick was less hospitable. The people were disturbed by the appearance of American Indians at Anicinabe and upset over the armed attempt to settle local grievances. They impeached their young chief, opting again for the steady counsel of Andy Keewatin. Tommy became a consultant on mercury pollution matters, his salary paid through the National Indian Brotherhood.

Passions raised by the park occupation had, as Mayor Davidson observed, beneficial spinoffs. Aside

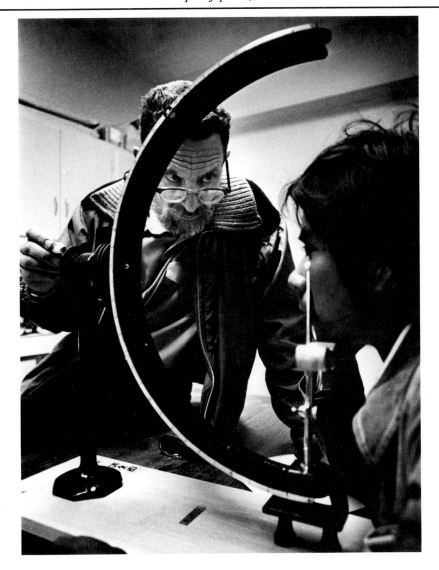

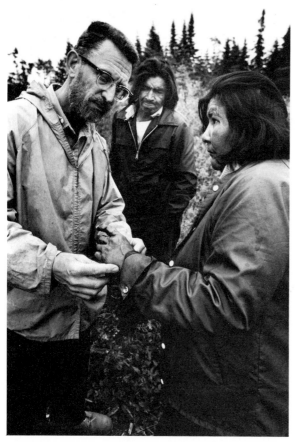

Wounds being treated by Dr. Peter Newberry.

from concentrating public attention on the Indian problems and forcing lethargic governments to respond, if only tokenly, there were positive gains. Demonstrating that their concern was not fleeting, the Quakers co-operated with the Indian Brotherhood and dispatched a doctor to Grassy Narrows to study the medical impact of mercury on the band.

Dr. Peter Newberry, a fifty-year-old native of South Africa, had retired in 1973 after nearly twenty years as a physician with the Royal Canadian Air Force. His detached analysis of mercury's effects on Grassy rapidly evolved into a deep commitment to help the people stabilize what was left of their community.

The bearded doctor read everything he could find on the symptoms of mercury poisoning and launched tests which the literature suggested for detection of signs. What he found startled and disturbed him. Among seventeen volunteers, all heavy fish eaters, he discovered at least one symptom in each of fifteen persons. He was convinced he was reading the early signs of Minamata Disease.

"My tests have shown up a surprisingly high incidence of impairment of peripheral vision," the physician said. Equally upsetting was the physical disintegration caused by other forces. Violent death was occurring almost monthly during the autumn and winter of 1974-75.

The band council met several times to discuss the violence, but was unable to find answers. "We just can't cope with it," said Andy Keewatin. "We have got to have the police come in here."

The Ontario Provincial Police parked a mobile office on the outskirts of the reserve and moved four men into the Grassy Narrows detachment. Many of the people resented the patrols by the black and white police vehicles, but the officers handled family quarrels and drunken episodes with tact and compassion. Gradually, the police were accepted and the violence tapered off. "I think we have saved a few lives," OPP Corporal Bill Bailey noted.

Government officials and politicians continued to deny the existence of Minamata Disease in northwestern Ontario, persisting in attributing the native's unusual behavior to alcohol, rather than mercury. There was still no proof that mercury was a serious health threat, they said.

Down the English River near Whitedog, not far from the Cariboo Dam, Adolph Kizikas had for years fished without concern of personal harm. But lately he had been worried by the strange sickness that had been affecting his cats, fed on scraps and small fish tossed their way. They had been disappearing, one by one, or staggering and growling, as if intoxicated. He found two drowned in a creek. In the autumn of 1974, his sixth cat fell victim to the malady, lying low and emitting a guttural growl that built to a scream, whirling and jumping in the air for as long as two hours at a time. The cat's mouth filled with frothing saliva and it urinated uncontrollably.

The sickness lasted through the winter and caught the attention of Jill Torrie, a young fieldworker for the National Indian Brotherhood from Kenora. In February 1975, Adolph Kizikas' cat was

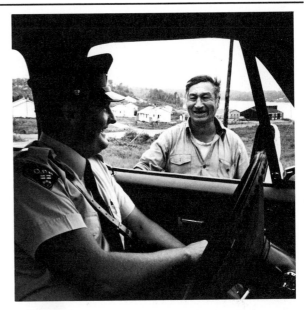

Police patrol.

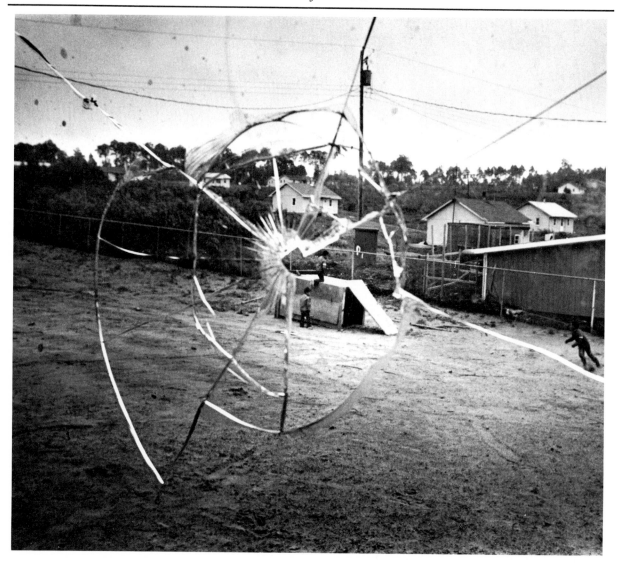

destroyed and its carcass sent to Toronto for analysis. Further studies were conducted in Japan and Michigan. The results were conclusive: the cat was a victim of Minamata Disease.

Tests on the Whitedog cat, as it came to be called, revealed 16.4 parts per million of mercury in its brain and an astonishing 392 ppm in its fur. Cats similarly affected in Minamata twenty years earlier averaged 11.8 ppm in the brain and only 45.8 ppm in fur.

A month later, a cat from Grassy Narrows was destroyed and tests conducted, with lower recordings but equally alarming results — a brain level of 6.9 ppm and fur level of 45.8 ppm.

Dr. Tadao Takeuchi, a pathologist at Kumamoto University, north of Minamata, told Aileen Smith his verdict on samples from the Whitedog cat: "There is no doubt that the occurrence of Minamata Disease in cats in the Indian reserve exists. I wish to study the autopsy cases of men in the near future."

Despite the tentative evidence offered by the animals of both reserves, federal and provincial medical authorities were unmoved. From blood tests taken among residents in January and February 1975, a federal official concluded there was "no suggestion" that mercury was affecting health.

In form letters sent to the Indians in March, Peter J. Connop, zone director of the federal medical services branch, suggested the residents simply "reduce" their fish intake.

"Most of the band members have mercury levels which are higher than the people living in Southern Ontario who do not eat very much fish," he wrote, "but this is to be expected and the mercury level does vary from person to person without necessarily having any effect on their health. We consider your mercury level to be in the range of measurements which would not affect your health.

"We realize that this matter of mercury in fish is a difficult one to understand and the experts are still learning more about mercury and its effects, but it is also important to remember that to keep healthy it is necessary to eat balanced meals which contain some meat or fish as well as starchy foods such as bread, and fats such as margarine or butter."

The National Indian Brotherhood branded the letter "an open invitation to a full-scale mercury poisoning disaster."

The letter was an embarrassment to Frank Miller, Ontario's health minister, who promised the Legislature it would not be sent out again. In an effort to explain it, he compared it to the warning carried on cigarette packages about the dangers of smoking. The letter simply advised Indians who persisted in eating fish the least damaging way of doing it.

Miller, a Muskoka resort operator in private life, was in an awkward position on the mercury issue, compelled as health minister to warn people against eating fish bearing more than .5 ppm of mercury while unable to prevent sportsmen and Indians from fishing the polluted waterways and eating their catches. "I'm tired of taking the flak for something on which I only give advice," he complained publicly.

In a sense, Miller epitomized the government's confusion, unable to legitimize the continued sports use of the English-Wabigoon chain, yet refusing to insist on its closure; conscious of the potential threat of mercury poisoning, yet unconvinced that damage had already been caused. Miller expressed a concern for the health of the people at Grassy and Whitedog, but said, "apparently in the area it isn't a burning issue."

"It is with the activists," he added, "who have been trying to make the Indians aware that it's dangerous to eat the fish. But we are dealing with a centuries-old habit, and it isn't easily changed, no matter how hard we try. The problem is real. We've been tackling it. But it's something like playing with jelly."

Miller said his experience in dealing with the mercury dilemma had taught him the difficulty in solving Indian problems. "And I don't mean that in a derogatory way. I mean we simply are not able to understand how to communicate and how to solve the problems of the Indians. We think we do. We go up there on a two- or three-day tour and come back and say 'we'll do this, or we'll do that' to resolve it. But we don't resolve it."

Miller was one of the more engaging members of the Davis cabinet, a seemingly compassionate man with a ready smile and a candor unusual among politicians, but he was burned when in the Legislature he later tried to put the mercury crisis in perspective by once again using the cigarette-smoking analogy. He said that many people die as a consequence of their own faulty decisions, and gave

eating poisoned fish, driving without a seat belt or smoking cigarettes as examples. The *Globe and Mail* published his remarks and responded with a damning editorial cartoon of two Indians carrying a comatose friend to the health minister's desk. "Mercury, eh?" the caricature of Miller was saying. "Tell him to use his seat belt, cut out smoking and get plenty of exercise." In a letter to the newspaper Miller explained his remark was prompted by "the frustration I felt about the unnecessary loss of life in other ways in Ontario. Every life we can save is precious. We are doing much now for the Indians — and I promise to continue. At the same time, many non-Indian people who are quite properly concerned about mercury and its effects on the Indians are needlessly dying because they feel government has no right to tell them not to smoke, drink, or drive without seat belts."

Meanwhile, tensions between whites and Indians from all reserves in the Kenora district were being further heightened by the appearance of a book entitled *Bended Elbow,* written by a local housewife who bitterly attacked the Indians for dragging the town's name into an international spotlight.

"I love this town," wrote Eleanor Jacobson in her paperback defence of Kenora, a small book filled with pictures of drunken Indians fighting, fornicating or just lying around. "I was born and raised here. But I'm ashamed to go downtown. Just what do you think the tourists think when they see these Indians relieving themselves of urine on the sidewalks in broad daylight! You can just imagine!"

The Jacobson book was vigorously attacked and

**I feel certain that as examinations continue,
they will eventually find a person with Minamata Disease. . . .
Please don't repeat the mistake we made in Japan.** *Dr. Masazumi Harada*

defended, dramatizing the division in the town. One reader, identifying herself as a "ripped-off taxpayer", told the local newspaper it was about time someone laid out the facts, regardless how sordid. Another dismissed the book as a "wedge between people."

Kenora was earmarked for even more unwanted attention. The letter sent by Marion Lamm to Eugene and Aileen Smith had set in motion a kind of international environmental pact between the Minamata victims and the Indians of Grassy Narrows and Whitedog. Aileen Smith's 1974 visit to Kenora had provided her with information she could give the Japanese scientists. Dr. Jun Ui, a professor of urban engineering at Tokyo University, and Dr. Masazumi Harada of Kumamoto University, a leading diagnostician of Minamata Disease, decided to see for themselves. They examined about twenty persons on the two reserves in March 1975.

"I found symptoms that can be found with methyl mercury poisoning," Harada reported to a seminar at the University of Toronto. "I feel certain that as examinations continue, they will eventually find a person with Minamata Disease. To we Japanese, who have made various mistakes in pollution, this situation is very shocking. Please don't repeat the mistakes we made in Japan."

Dr. Ui warned, "If you don't start action you will have a more serious result than we had."

During a visit to Ottawa, they quizzed federal officials about testing measures and learned, for the first time, that cats fed fish from Clay Lake had developed Minamata Disease. The tests had never

been disclosed to the people of Grassy Narrows and Whitedog.

"Canadian politicians have been incredibly apathetic," Aileen Smith commented. "I think it comes from a belief that it will not become a blatant enough epidemic where the press can go in there and photograph people who are having horrible convulsions, where it will become a big scandal.

"They believe it can be contained. But there is an absurdity in the thought that if they don't do something it will somehow go away.

"Actually, they've spent more money trying to cover up the issue than if they had relocated the camp operators on different lakes and said the Indians would receive food shipments."

She said the bureaucratic parallels between the Kenora district and Minamata were "unbelievable".

"The way the government reacted, the way the companies are [unaffected by] direct criticism. To say that the Kenora area is equal to Minamata, well, there's no epidemic yet. But as far as the government reaction is concerned, there are incredible parallels.

"The Canadian government, the Canadian people, should not repeat the mistakes of the Japanese people. They should initiate a policy that does not allow, economically, the fish to be consumed. It's really that simple. Yelling and being shocked by an outbreak is too late."

On their return to Japan, the scientists relayed to the victims of Minamata Disease what they had learned during the Canadian tour. Within weeks, Chief Andy Keewatin of Grassy Narrows and Chief

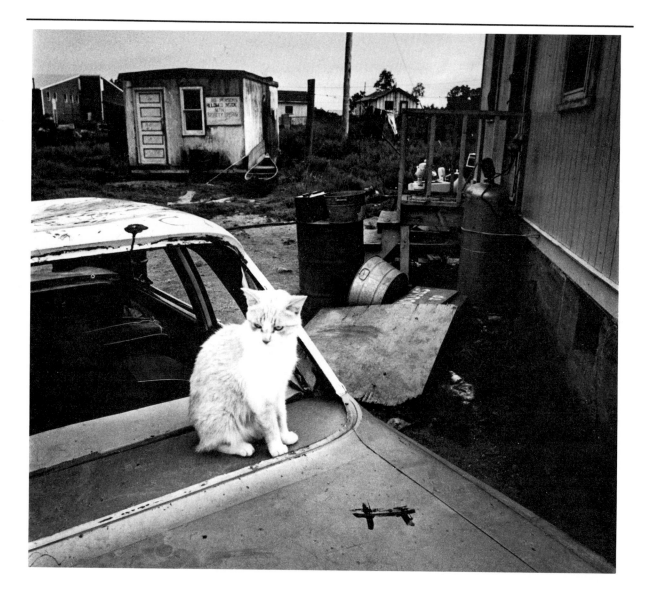

We cannot think of your problem as a stranger's problem.
Tsuginori Hamamoto

Roy McDonald of Whitedog received a letter from Tsuginori Hamamoto, of the Minamata Disease Patients' Alliance.

"We cannot think of your problem as a stranger's problem," he wrote. "We Minamata Disease patients, as victims of Japan's industry and government and capitalists, have these several decades been discriminated [against] by the world around us and have tasted poverty and physical and mental suffering.

"The real dread of mercury can only be understood by those who have had their bodies made bad, and . . . their families. And if you rely on [the company], the central government or the provincial government — they will do nothing for you.

"There is no other way to open up the road to help but for you . . . to stand and speak your suffering and the anxiety of your sickness to many people. After eating fish for a long time — and before you realize it — mercury makes your bodies sick, and your hands and feet . . . unable to move, and not just become numb, paralyzed and have convulsions, but when bad, in one night, can make all of the body no good. It is not just a few who die.

"We invite you . . . to Minamata, because we want you to see what the dread of mercury is. It will be a blessing if our long years of suffering can help you in even one single way. We feel you will understand the dreadfulness of the pouring out of poisons and pollution that is spreading over this earth. If we can help you in changing the anxiety that you have in your hearts in even one single way — it will be good."

A delegation was formed. The federal government and the National Indian Brotherhood agreed to fund transportation for Andy Keewatin, Tommy Keesick and Bill Fobister from Grassy, Tony Henry and Jack Kent from Whitedog, and Jill Torrie, the fieldworker from the National Indian Brotherhood. Dr. Peter Newberry would go along at the expense of the Minamata victims. Barney Lamm would also attend; he paid his own way.

Andy Keewatin said, "We want to see what shape the people are in over there. Maybe we can understand a little from them."

8

To Minamata

The traditional Japanese party at the downtown Tokyo restaurant was intended to be a happy occasion, a welcome for the Indians from Canada. But just as everyone seated themselves around the low table to feast on raw fish, shrimp, octopus and rice, one of the hostesses suffered an attack of the unpredictable disease.

The tips of her fingers of her left hand buckled under a debilitating cramp that began travelling up her arm. She tried to maintain a smile for her guests, but the pain crippled her and two young people hastened to massage her racked arm muscles and crooked fingers. She fell back and muffled her cries as the shock hit her shoulder. Tears welled up in her eyes.

"That's one of the symptoms," someone told the Indians, who watched with embarrassment and worry.

As the pain subsided, the woman resumed her place at the table, bowing and apologizing through a young interpreter for the untimely interruption. She blushed self-consciously, but extended her hand to show the involuntary tremors, the vestiges of the attack. The Indians stared at her quivering fingers and realized they were looking at Minamata Disease, the crippler and killer they had journeyed halfway around the world to see and to learn about.

The film they were shown on their arrival in Japan, in July of 1975, was a trilogy on the devastation caused by mercury pollution from the giant Chisso Corporation on Minamata Bay. A graphic portrayal of human suffering, it provoked shock and anger. From the screen, the eyes of a young girl,

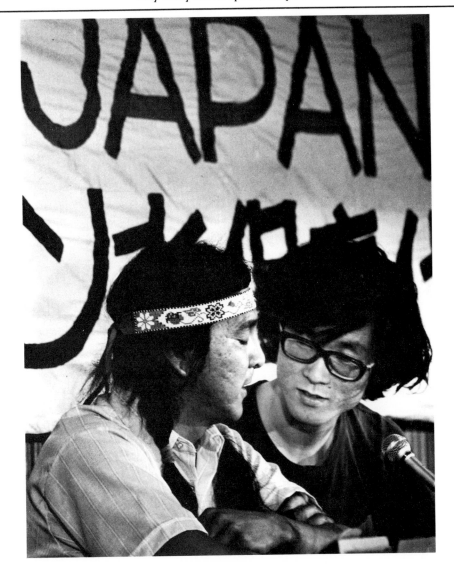

perhaps twelve or thirteen years old, stared emptily. She wrung her deformed hands, while her mother told the interviewer of the strange disease that had made her this way.

"Our cats seemed to go mad and run amuck in the room," the mother explained. "We covered ourselves with a comforter to avoid getting hurt. Some cats jumped in the sea and came home soaking wet. Our five cats died, one after another."

"Then, she was suddenly attacked by the disease." The girl's head rolled and eyes searched vainly for meaning in her mother's words and gestures. "When she cried, she sounded like the cats. We thought she had contracted the disease from them. After that, my family was shunned, as if it had an infectious disease."

In the darkened amphitheater, the Indian leaders shuddered, recalling the death of cats at Grassy and Whitedog, and the secret government tests on cats fed fish from Clay Lake. Those cats, too, had performed a strange dance of death, staggering, salivating, convulsing and dying to the sounds of their own squeals.

In another of the film's scenes, a man driven to premature old age by the mercury poison in his brain and nervous system writhed on the floor. His eyes bulged and his emaciated lips moved, but he was unable to speak. The voice of a doctor told the audience: "I think he is trying to say 'Help me. Help me'."

"It is like something out of Hollywood," Tommy Keesick said. "A horror movie." He said that the terrible questions raised by the film must be answered.

The film told of government lethargy and Chisso's resistance to any public scrutiny of the pollution problem. One early researcher, a scientist from Kumamoto University, related how he and a colleague were prevented from gathering samples near the chemical plant to test their theory that Chisso was the polluter.

"They wouldn't let us in, so we trespassed beyond the fence. We were caught by a guard and ordered to abandon the samples. Since we were accustomed to being honest, we gave them up, to our regret. In elucidating the cause [of the pollution] Chisso Corporation has never shown a co-operative attitude."

Barney Lamm smiled wryly, recalling the sudden appearance of a fence at the chemical plant back in Dryden soon after his unannounced visit there in 1970.

The film also talked about the mounting pressure on Chisso as the extent of the environmental and human damage became apparent, how the president of Chisso eventually conceded that the company had a moral — though not a legal — responsibility. His concession was not unlike the one made later by the president of the Dryden pulp and paper operations.

A Chisso worker told of the haphazard handling of mercury inside the plant; the company's attitude was so casual that he "became numb to the danger of it." He explained, "After Minamata Disease broke out, the company told us to discharge the mercury at night or to clean the ditch where mercury was

**We should work together to try to show the government,
the polluters, that we are the ones who are suffering, not them.**
Bill Fobister

discharged. We hid the fact that mercury waste was always discarded."

Bill Fobister, a sensitive man who craved solutions to the problems confronting his people back at Grassy Narrows, commented, "It seems to me that we are in the same position. They are polluting our livelihood and destroying our economy. So we have the same problem and we should work together to try to show the government, the polluters, that we are the ones who are suffering, not them."

Tommy Keesick, less patient after five years of inaction, suggested that "one has to be a little radical to get things done."

"Any expression on our return [to Canada] lies in the hands of the government officials," the young Ojibway "warrior" warned. "If they still do not want to co-operate or get off their high horse and listen to the oppressed people, then more serious confrontations will be held. It will be time that native people across Canada will have only one alternative, and that is to become radical. If radical measures are the only ones left, then they should be taken."

Andy Keewatin worried about his colleague's remarks, mindful of the backlash to last summer's occupation of Anicinabe Park. "You don't have to be militant to prove something," said the chief. The Japanese hosts nodded approvingly at Tommy's words, knowingly at Andy's.

"Among the people of Minamata," explained Aileen Smith, serving as tour guide and interpreter, "there was always a belief the government would be fair and the government had the knowledge and ability to deal with the problems thoroughly and properly. But it was only by being disillusioned repeatedly that finally, in 1969, some of the victims took Chisso to court."

The people had accepted disillusionment for too long, for many reasons. Chisso represented prosperity for Minamata. The forerunner of the giant corporation built a factory in the town in 1907 and as it grew, so did the community. In the years leading up to the Second World War and in the years of reconstruction following the conflict, Chisso first prospered through its production of fertilizer and carbide, then through meeting the growing demand for plastics and chemical compounds.

In 1932, Chisso began producing acetaldehyde, using mercury as a catalyst in the process. Acetaldehyde was vital to the manufacture of plastics, some drugs and perfumes, a market that boomed in the post-war years. As the sale of acetaldehyde from Minamata accelerated, so did the incidence of environmental damage. Fish began floating to the surface of the bay and cats began their dances of death. In April 1956, the first recognized case of Minamata Disease was admitted to Chisso's factory hospital. In the ensuing years, more than a hundred persons would die from the disease and as many as ten thousand would suffer varying degrees of injury, from numbness of extremities to mental retardation and blindness. (The official toll of victims was smaller. As of 1974 only 798 were considered "verified" victims; that is, cases of Minamata Disease confirmed by the board of physicians the state had appointed to determine who was a true victim. Another 2,800 had applied for verification.)

Despite an "outbreak" of the disease that raged through the late-1950s and early-1960s, Chisso continued to discharge mercury with its sewage until 1968 and persistently refused to acknowledge any legal responsibility to the victims of its actions. Then, the patients began to channel their grief into legal actions and protests. They staged sit-ins and, at one point, bought stock in the corporation in order to attend and disrupt stockholders' meetings with their demands for compensation. A leader of the cause was Teruo Kawamoto, a courageous and flamboyant activist, a verified victim himself, who was driven by the conviction that face-to-face confrontation with Chisso executives would force them to compensate victims of the disease. At the height of the protests, he jammed the gates of Chisso with his slight body for five hours in a symbolic gesture of his unshakable resolve.

In 1973, twenty-nine families, representing forty-five victims of Minamata Disease, won their battle fought in the streets and the courts. The legal judgment initially cost Chisso $3.2 million and eventually more than $80 million in settlements.

The judge ruled: *"The defendant's plant discharged acetaldehyde waste water with negligence at all times, and even though the quality and content of the waste water of the defendant's plant satisfied statutory limitations and administrative standards, and even if the treatment methods it employed were superior to those taken at the work yards of other companies in the same industry . . . the defendant cannot escape from the liability of negligence."*

Chisso was ordered to pay from ninety dollars a month to those with minor afflictions, to sixty-eight thousand dollars to survivors, family members who had endured irreparable physical and emotional suffering.

The Japanese were convinced that militancy had brought them some retribution, if only in monetary terms, and they made sure that their Indian guests from North America got the message.

In the pitching sightseeing bus that carried them to Minamata Bay, Tsuginori Hamamoto, himself crippled by mercury, advised his guests to become more militant or invite further abuse from industry and authorities back in Canada. "With the knowledge you get from this visit," his voice crackled over the loudspeaker, "you can confront the company and the government. Unless you realize this, the trip is pointless." In a way, the trip to Japan in itself was a step toward militancy, a physical demonstration of resolve and solidarity by the five Indians and their white travelling companions.

The destination of the bumpy ride through the baked countryside of Kyushu Prefecture was the city by the bay of the Shiranui Sea and neighboring fishing villages. Hamamoto, whose sister was also crippled and whose parents had died from mercury poisoning, took the opportunity to tell the visitors, "The world will become worse and worse unless people like you take a stand."

"Although we patients are not radical," he said, "we finally had to take a very stringent stand in order to save ourselves. We had never heard of demonstrations, trials, court action. But we were cornered into it. There was no way we were able to save ourselves. By our action, the government was forced to admit there was a problem and forced to try to do something about it."

As the bus neared Minamata, teacher Hiroshi Oshimure took the microphone next. "In a way," he said, "one can say Chisso brought civilization, scientific civilization to Minamata. And in the measure that such civilization can bring happiness, perhaps Chisso did bring this kind of happiness."

"However," Oshimure continued, "this civilization brought about pollution and the victimization of us Minamata citizens. It was only after the victims rose up and pointed it out that it was made public that Chisso was responsible for the pollution...

"The truth was made clear not by the government, nor industry, nor scientists, nor medical people, nor lawyers, but by the people of Minamata themselves. I think this is true in other areas. I believe in Canada, also, that it is not only through science that this truth can be made clear. It will be through the people themselves."

There was a certain irony, a bizarre twist of the calendar, to the timing of the Indians' visit. Elsewhere, other North American visitors were arriving in Okinawa, to attend the opening of Expo '75, a world's fair dedicated to the preservation of the world's marine environment.

"Mother sea, who used to be beautiful, so brilliant in her green dress under the radiant sun, is becoming sick from the pollution caused by the indiscriminate dumping of industrial waste beyond the ocean's capacity for natural purification," visitors to Expo were told. "Man must awaken to this crisis. Man must reflect on past errors...." Perhaps the world's fair should have been held in Minamata.

The bus trip to Minamata was long and hot, the bus crowded, cramped and sweaty. But a cheerful atmosphere prevailed as the Indians got to know their hosts. They joked about their facial similarities and one girl combed Tommy Keesick's thick black hair. Despite his revolutionary rhetoric, he was a charmer, and he captivated both the Japanese people and the Japanese press.

A small welcoming committee greeted the visitors on their arrival in Minamata at the end of the three-hour bus ride and treated them to a relaxing, informal dinner of fish and shellfish from the Shiranui Sea. The tour would begin the next day, when the devastating and insidious consequences of industrial pollution would be translated from Japanese to Ojibway in human terms.

"They come, they come," thirteen-year-old Takako Isayama managed to slur as the Indians visited her home. She let out a happy cry and her twisted limbs shook with excitement as, one by one, they said hello and touched her. "She can talk, but only a few words," they were told. "She understands what you are saying."

Takako was one of the forty children born during the Minamata Disease outbreak with congenital defects, which were later traced to their mothers' heavy fish consumption throughout pregnancy. The mercury had penetrated the placental barrier and accumulated in the wombs of the mothers, attacking

the unborn children, causing stillbirths and deformities. Of the original forty, at least seven had
subsequently died, the most recent victim a twenty-
four-year-old man who strangled because of his
increasing difficulty in swallowing.

Unlike Takako, who could enjoy her life at
home to some degree, most of the survivors spent
their lives in the nursing home at Meisuien, one of
the first stops on the Ojibways' tour. Chizuri
Nakama was there. Chizuri would always be there,
a few minutes' drive from the Chisso plant.

Eighteen-year-old Chizuri had the mind of an
infant. She was lying on a mat, surrounded by
others in wheelchairs, as the Indians entered the
bright nursery. Again, they heard the happy wail
and saw the trembling limbs, the unco-ordinated
eyes searching for the visitors. Tommy Keesick knelt
beside her.

"My name is Tommy," he said. "If I get your
name I will write a letter to you." The cry. "Maybe
she does not understand," Tommy commented to a
staff member, "but she is my sister from a long way
away."

"She says yes," he was told. "She can say yes, no,
but she cannot say much more."

A doctor told the visitors that "all the parents
had light symptoms of Minamata Disease, but it
came out very acutely in the children. The legs that
are crossed like that," he said, pointing to Chizuri's
tangled limbs, "that is seen very often in Minamata
Disease."

The Indians were told it was vital that contaminated fish not be eaten, especially by pregnant
women. "If they don't keep a close watch on it, it is
possible to get acute Minamata Disease, like this."

"It seems to me such a tragedy," said Dr. Peter
Newberry. "All that suffering, which really can't be
alleviated, and the expense of providing this beautiful hospital. It could have been avoided at a fraction
of the cost by interrupting the pollution as soon as
people became aware it was there."

"The main benefit of this trip," he said, "is that
the Indian people who have come here will be convinced at a gut level of the danger of eating
contaminated fish and, hopefully, will be able to get
this gut message across to the people of Grassy and
Whitedog."

The tour circled the sprawling Chisso plant and
stopped near a landfill site north of the factory.
Aileen Smith explained that the company had for a
time stopped dumping its effluent into the bay by
diverting it into a channel flowing directly to the
Shiranui Sea. But the mercury simply spread along
the coast, contaminating more fish and poisoning
more people. The experimental outfall and its
deadly sludge was buried and the bay once again
became the cesspool.

On their tour of the shoreline, aboard fishing
boats which were taking them to visit villages up
and down the coast, the North Americans saw
another mad experiment. It was a net, stretched
roughly two thousand feet across the mouth of
Minamata Bay, designed, presumably, to keep poisoned fish in and pure fish out. But in the center,
there was a gaping hole which allowed boats and
fish in and out.

Andy Keewatin at Chisso dump site, Japan, 1975.

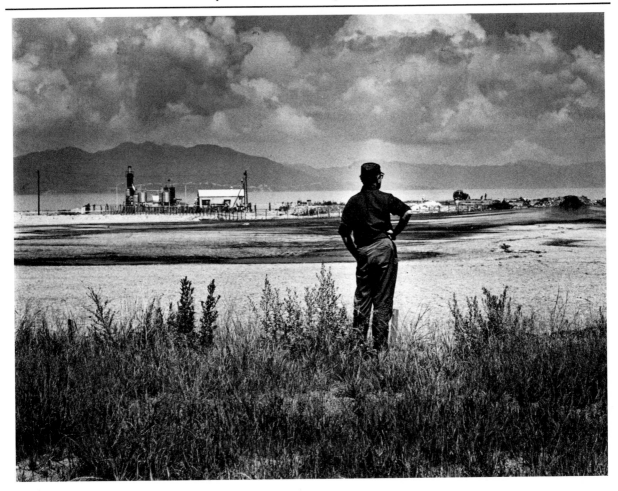

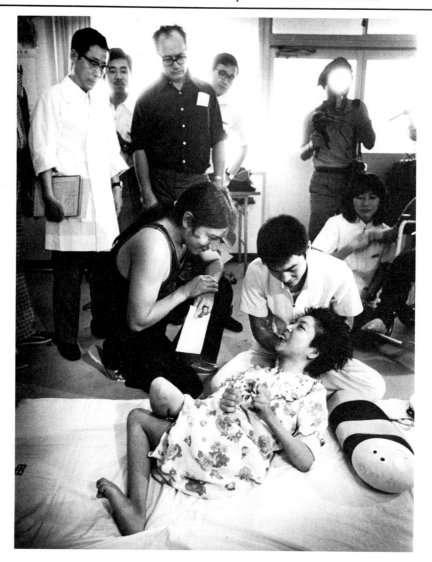

122

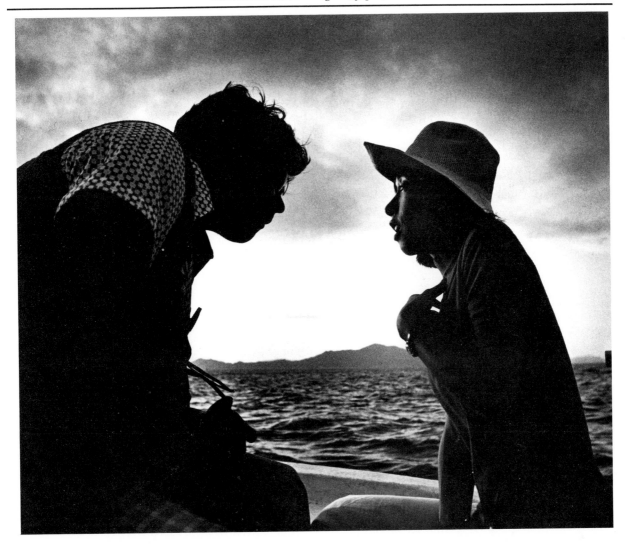

The protective net, Minamata Bay, 1975.

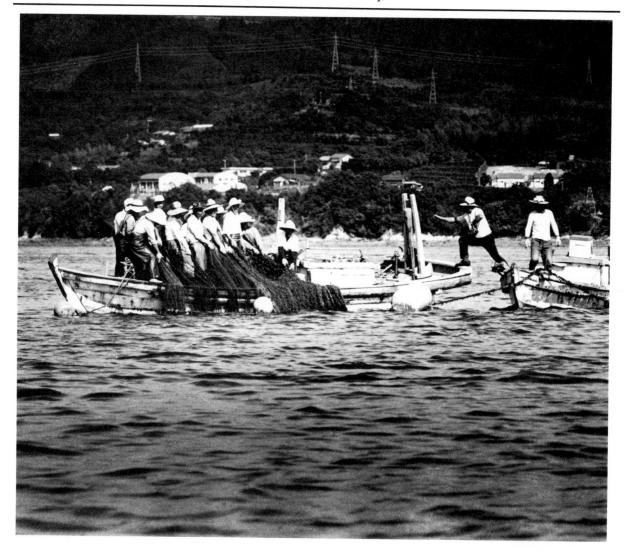

By the time you see an acute,
indisputable case of Minamata Disease, it is too late.
Dr. Masazumi Harada

In the village of Meshima, the wives of fishermen rushed for their cameras as the tourists arrived at their doors. They photographed the Indians, but appeared more interested in the tall, round-eyed whites, a novelty in these parts. The travellers exchanged polite pleasantries, then headed for the home of sixteen-year-old Masazumi Kosaki.

They crowded into his livingroom — Indians, interested villagers, print and television journalists — and Masazumi was helped in by his father, Teruo. The boy was a congenital victim, crippled from birth. He sat on the floor, rocking with his head down, his hands twisted in front of him, saliva dripping from his chin. Someone turned on TV floodlights and Masazumi winced. "Lights bother his eyes," his father explained through an interpreter, and the lights were turned off.

"He loves to watch television," said Teruo Kosaki. "That's the way he spends his time. He can't walk, so he goes on a wheelchair. A teacher comes in twice a week to the home. [Masazumi] can't speak, but he is very smart. He can hear everything. He is very smart."

"How do you feel about what has happened to your son?" the father was asked.

"It is a hatred," he replied. "A kind of feeling we can't express in words."

"Do you still eat fish?"

"Yes," he said. "Without eating the fish, we cannot live."

"He is just like us," remarked Andy Keewatin, although later he would admit that he was unprepared for the volume of seafood in the Japanese diet.

"I'll tell you one thing," the chief said during one of the few quiet interludes in the busy schedule. "They eat a lot more fish than we do."

That fact has probably saved many Canadian lives, Dr. Newberry observed. "I am convinced there are a number of people at Grassy and Whitedog with early signs of Minamata Disease, and I am puzzled that it is not more apparent. The most likely explanation is that they don't eat quite as much fish as the Japanese fishermen, and this is helped by the fact their intake tends to be seasonal."

In the days that followed, the Indians visited the homes of other victims, enjoyed an evening fishing trip on the Shiranui Sea and, before leaving Minamata, were invited as guests to a town meeting held in their honor.

Hardly a breeze entered through the open windows of the town hall. Outside, children scrambled after noisy cicadas, competing with the noise of whirring electric fans for the attention of the townspeople, primarily members of afflicted families, who sat on mats, fanning themselves.

Dr. Masazumi Harada, the pioneer in Minamata Disease diagnosis, explained the reason for exposing the Indians to "the suffering of Minamata." He said it was an early warning exercise to prevent suffering in Grassy Narrows and Whitedog.

"By the time you see an acute, indisputable case of Minamata Disease," he said, "it is too late. An outbreak has already occurred. We must not repeat this situation again. There is proof enough that people have already been affected by mercury poisoning in Canada." He encouraged the people of

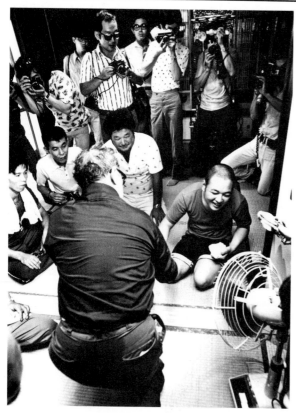

Andy Keewatin visiting the Kosaki home, Japan, 1975.

Minamata to lend the Indians their support. "You were alone twenty years ago," he said. "They, the Indians, are exactly in the same position you were in."

Tsuginori Hamamoto, as chairman of the Minamata Disease Patients' Alliance, repeated his plea for action. "We thought this kind of tragedy would not be seen anywhere else in the world," he said. "When Dr. Harada told us of the similarity of our situations, it made us very angry. Now there is pollution in Canada, and pollution is spreading all over the world. We cannot relax. From Canada, from Minamata, let us join and fight together."

Chief Andy Keewatin thanked the people of Minamata for their kindness, then Tommy Keesick had his say: "The government, I hope, will not repeat the mistake made here. I hope three hundred of us don't have to die before the government finally acts."

Tommy promised that "more serious confrontation will be held elsewhere in Canada, and this includes the Indian people in the United States." He said his wife was carrying his child and vowed, "If I detect any physical defect in my child when it is born, if it is blind or deaf, believe me I will go to all the ultimate extreme battles necessary."

There was cautious applause from the Japanese audience, and Peter Newberry was moved to explain.

"Our hearts have been torn and our minds baffled at the suffering we have seen in your homes," he said to the hushed crowd. "I have known Tommy as a brother, and I can understand the views he has

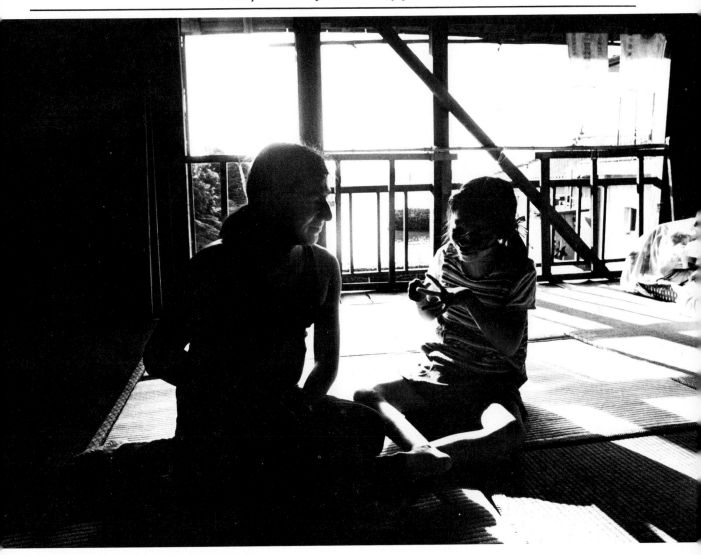

A visit with Jitsuko Tanaka, a Minamata victim (extreme left). Among the Canadian visitors are Bill Fobister, viewing a picture of Jitsuko before she was crippled, Tommy Keesick to his right, and Andy Keewatin (fourth from the left).

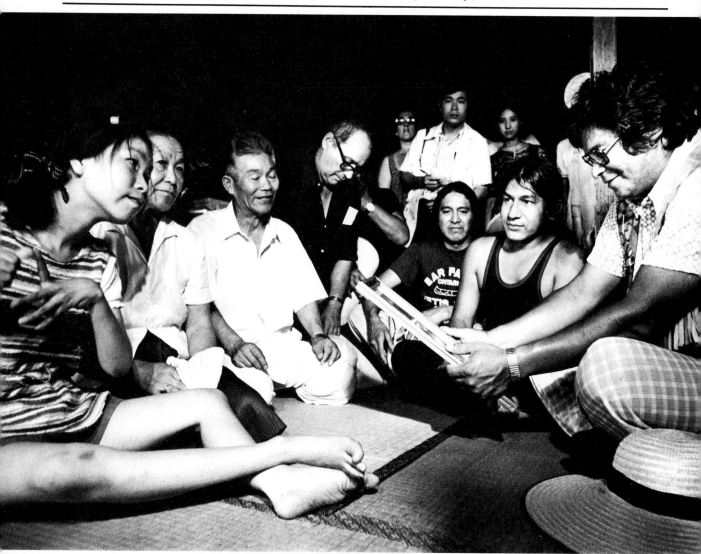

expressed. However, they are caused by an anguish in his heart."

The Quaker doctor said there are times when people must take direct action to correct injustices, "but we must strive with all the power we have to avoid violence in these confrontations."

"This beautiful country which you have, and the beautiful country my brothers have in Canada, we must leave for our children in the condition that we find it. Industry is the life blood of our society, but we must not let it walk recklessly over that society...."

Barney Lamm was also asked to speak and applauded the people of Minamata for the reception and hospitality shown to "my boys." As former employer of most of the Indian leaders on the tour, he retained his paternalistic attitude toward them. But they did not take exception to his remarks.

Outside the hall, Barney cited financial, personal and moral involvement as reasons enough for him to be there. But, even with the knowledge about mercury he had accumulated in the intervening five years, he was dumbfounded by the sights he had witnessed, on film and in person.

"I am here because I wanted to see first hand what things looked like here, to see how they compare with our problems at Grassy and Whitedog. I wanted to see the early signs in the victims, how they looked and how they acted and what effect it had on them.

"There is no question in my mind that there are people at Grassy and Whitedog who have been hurt by the poisoning. Every day there seem to be more

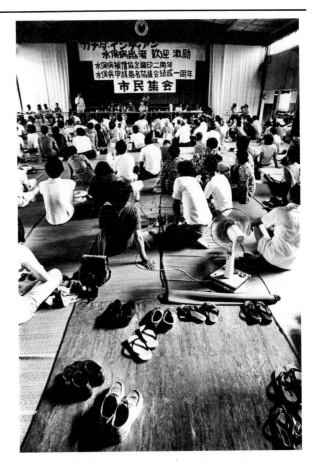

A town hall meeting for the Canadian visitors, Minamata, 1975.

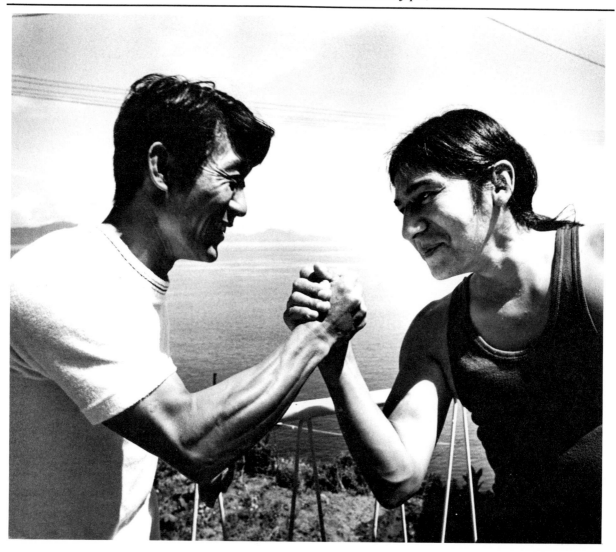

Keesick teaches Kawamoto the "radical" handshake, Japan, 1975.

definite signs. From the cats that died, they confirmed it was mercury poisoning, Minamata Disease. So, there's no question in my mind that we are on the verge of a minor 'Minamata.' It is there.

"Sure, I have a financial interest in being here. There's no question about it. But I have probably more of a personal concern than most people. The people who are being affected at Grassy and Whitedog all worked for us. The younger generation that's there were born there and grew up there. These are our friends and it's real important to us that something be done."

Teruo Kawamoto, the man who had led the struggle for compensation from Chisso, also addressed the audience and the Indian guests.

"Man's progress and the precedent of industry's pursuit of profit is the cause of our sad meeting," he said. "Pollution seems to cover the whole of our earth and is on the way to destroying both our bodies and spirit.

"Geographically, Canada and Japan are distant countries. But though we live in different countries, we share the same agony, caused by the mercury discharge from industry.

"We are responsible for ourselves and for our children and the ones who are coming on. Mother Nature and the surroundings are not anybody's belonging. Much more, they are not for anybody to possess exclusively. We have a right to have the blessings and responsibility to protect them, as nature gives grace to men equally."

On the way back through Kumamoto, the Indians stopped by the university for tests by Dr. Harada. There were only suggestive signs, nothing definite, that they might be suffering early stages of mercury poisoning. They were also taken to a private audience with Issei Sawada, governor of Kumamoto Prefecture, who admitted his government was not doing enough, "but we are trying harder, so that this terrible situation does not happen again." They were amazed by this experience.

"I have been here a few days and already I have seen the governor," remarked Jack Kent, one of the councillors from Whitedog. "He is thousands of miles away. But back home, I haven't seen the government in my life. That proves their government is doing something."

Tony Henry, of Whitedog, expressed it most simply: "We, the Canadian Indian, have never experienced such concern by a people."

9

Making Work

The alliance between the Indians and the people of Minamata was bound with the cement of common cause and led to further global travels in the summer of 1975, when a small band of scientists, headed by Dr. Masazumi Harada, made a second visit to Canada.

As a researcher at the University of Kumamoto medical school, Harada had worked extensively with Minamata Disease patients and was widely recognized as one of the leading diagnosticians of methyl mercury poisoning. He was anxious to follow up preliminary studies made the previous March and what he found confirmed earlier suspicions that Minamata Disease — at least in its initial stages — could be detected among the peoples of Grassy Narrows and Whitedog.

"The situation is clearly a reappearance of what happened in Minamata and Niigata, Japan," Harada warned in a summary of his startling findings.

From surveys on eighty-nine Indians, he discovered nineteen cases of disturbed eye movement, forty cases of impaired hearing, thirty-seven cases of sensory disturbance, sixteen cases of tunnel vision, twenty-one cases of tremor, twenty cases of reflex loss and eight cases of loss of balance.

"Glove-and-stocking sensory disturbance and paranoncentric contraction of visual field were found among those with high values of mercury concentration in blood and hair, and in some cases [the] same symptoms were found among their family members. In such cases, the influence of methyl mercury is suspected."

Natural Resources Minister Leo Bernier was

The situation is clearly a reappearance
of what happened in Minamata and Niigata, Japan.
Dr. Masazumi Harada

annoyed and embarrassed by the presence of the Japanese scientists in his home riding. Their visit was politically disruptive and, in a radio interview, he dismissed them as a "group of travelling troubadors."

The attitude was typical of the mood in Dryden, where the pulp and paper company's well-being was critical to the town.

The *Dryden Observer,* the local newspaper, stressed that Dryden was not Minamata and should not be linked with that Japanese city of death and tragedy. "Use of the name 'Dryden' in combination with 'Minamata Disease' and efforts to link mercury pollution in this area with that in Japan have been condemned by some medical authorities," the paper stated.

"The suggestion has been made that those individuals including writers and broadcasters using the term 'Dryden-Minamata Disease' be aware of the near-libellous nature of their act in linking the name of a town with something for which the town is not responsible . . . especially in view of the claims that no definite evidence of any 'disease' has been established."

The newspaper quoted the thesis of an American scientist that since mercury discharged in Japan was released in a methylated form, and mercury in Canada was released in an elemental state, its appearance in wildlife and humans might have differing effects. The Japanese scientists, however, detected no difference in the effect of mercury released from the Dryden mill, which was transformed to an organic state in the water, and

absorbed into the food chain.

Despite the embarrassment, Dryden could not escape Minamata, even after the departure of the Japanese scientists. In September of 1975, a small group of Minamata Disease patients, accompanied by Aileen Smith, arrived in Canada, to visit the two Indian reserves, the towns of Kenora and Dryden, and to present themselves as living evidence of mercury poisoning on the steps of the Ontario Legislature at Queen's Park in Toronto.

Although snubbed by a social planning committee in Kenora, the patients received a concerned reception from high school students who asked all kinds of questions about mercury in the environment and its effects on human beings. Its capacity to cripple was obvious in the form of Tsuginori Hamamoto, who hobbled about on canes or was wheeled to meetings in a wheelchair.

After a few days in the Kenora district, the Minamata patients, including Teruo Kawamoto, about forty Indians from Grassy Narrows and Whitedog, and a few white sympathizers, staged a symbolic march on Dryden, resplendent with banners and placards which exhorted mill operators to "Stop Dryden-Minamata Disease."

Hamamoto, wearing a white vest bearing anti-pollution slogans in Japanese, was wheeled through the gates of the sprawling pulp and paper installation by Marion Lamm, but they were told by a public relations officer they could not enter the chemical plant.

Over the years, the corporate face of the polluter had changed. Anglo-Canadian Pulp and Paper and a

**We must be prepared to shoulder our responsibility when it's clear what that is. . . .
Where there are proven cases of mercury poisoning,
or the so-called Minamata Disease, we will not take a legalistic approach. . . .**
Robert W. Billingsley

number of other Canadian holdings of the Reed empire were consolidated under the name of Reed Paper Holdings Ltd., which remained a subsidiary of Reed International Ltd. of Britain. In the process, Reed emerged as one of Canada's top sixty industries, with money or controlling interest in plants which produced a wide range of wood and pulp products, including kraft papers, furniture, fabrics, wallpaper and scores of accessories for home decoration.

Eighty-five per cent of Reed in Canada was owned by the British parent, which embraced in its family of companies a string of radio stations and newspapers, including the influential *Daily Mirror*. Reed International operated more than 400 companies, with concentration in the forest and mining sectors, in over forty countries around the globe.

Canadian directors of Reed Limited continued to include T. S. (Tom) Jones, former manager of the Dryden mill. Among the twenty-four officers and members of the board of directors was Renault St. Laurent, son of the late Louis St. Laurent, a former prime minister of Canada. Placed at the helm of the Canadian operations was Robert W. Billingsley, a brilliant young industrialist, yet to reach forty, who soared swiftly through the corporate hierarchy following his graduation from the University of Pennsylvania in 1960.

As president, Billingsley would set the pace for Reed in Canada. "Overall," he stated, "this company has a strong commitment to environmental protection, and currently has a number of programs either completed or under way. As well, we have an

internal management system which includes environmental protection as a key element in planning for all new projects."

Billingsley was given the job of answering for the company's past performance. He told an interviewer: "We must be prepared to shoulder our responsibility when it's clear what that is. . . . Where there are proven cases of mercury poisoning, or the so-called Minamata Disease, we will not take a legalistic approach. . . .

"I believe personally [that] as long as I am president of this company we must go beyond that and look at our moral and social responsibilities as people who live in Ontario and Canada, and must work there. I think our employees and our shareholders expect that."

The public outcry and broad media coverage given to the company's activities in northwestern Ontario, however, disturbed Reed's president and he told the Dryden District Chamber of Commerce that "undue panic and alarm have been created over the pollution problem."

Billingsley said the company was fully aware of public concern over the situation and had been co-operating with the provincial and federal governments to correct matters; for example, it had installed a new mercury-free system at the Dryden plant, at a cost of five million dollars. He repeated the oft-mentioned claim that "authorities have found no symptoms specifically attributable to methyl mercury poisioning in the peoples of the area."

"Unfortunately, the situation has been made

**Unfortunately,
the situation has been made more difficult by the often biased,
hysterical and, frankly, shoddy reporting by much of the media.**
Robert W. Billingsley

more difficult by the often biased, hysterical and, frankly, shoddy reporting by much of the media," he claimed.

Dryden mayor George Rowat, meanwhile, blamed Barney Lamm for a lot of the bad publicity. A crusty old politician with a tendency to speak his mind, Rowat complained that the Indians were being used by Lamm to make his personal legal case against Reed.

"Barney Lamm . . . should have been deported back to the United States years ago," he said. "Everything he has done he has done on somebody else's money. Barney Lamm never had the milk of human kindness to keep the Indian working. He has done more to discourage tourists from coming into Kenora and the English River chain than anyone can ever repair."

The mayor said he had heard a lot of people in Kenora had money invested in Barney's Ball Lake Lodge and lost it when the resort was closed. "I can't prove that," he admitted. "If you say that, and say that it's my opinion, I don't mind. You can say that."

Rowat also had little compassion for the situation in which the Indians found themselves: "If nothing had happened to the river, the Indians would be in the same position. The Indian has completely lost his incentive to work, because he has found an easier way. . . . At some place we've got to get back. Everyone has got to earn his own bread, one way or another."

The mayor said he was convinced the Indians had not been harmed by mercury, and Dryden only marginally so. "I don't believe it has hurt Dryden financially," he said. "I think people are hurt by the publicity that has come. It has settled on Dryden. But as far as Dryden is concerned, we don't even know about mercury, except they say it is there. We don't know of it affecting any of the population in the area."

Rowat said he resented that Dryden was being portrayed as the "fall guy" in the mercury episode, but conceded that the company could have done more to prevent pollution.

"There would have been a shooting war if someone had said 'We are going to shut you down.' The town's economy basically comes from the mill. You can talk about tourism, fishing, but if it wasn't for the mill being here, there wouldn't be a town."

"Everybody agrees it should be cleaned up, whether it's mercury pollution or any other pollution. How you do it is another thing. . . . Let's face it, they're a big company that doesn't give a damn for the town or the people. One thing about industry, and you can say I said it, they're just oriented toward the buck. The shareholders are more important than the people who do the work."

"My concern is the people of the town. But by the same token, more can be done by industry to alleviate problems of pollution. If we can send a rocket to the moon, I'm sure we can clean up pollution."

Rowat's words illustrated the unusual love-hate relationship between the town and the plant. The town smarted over its dirty name and wanted the company to clean up its act, but vigorously

Wilderness and industry, Dryden, 1976.

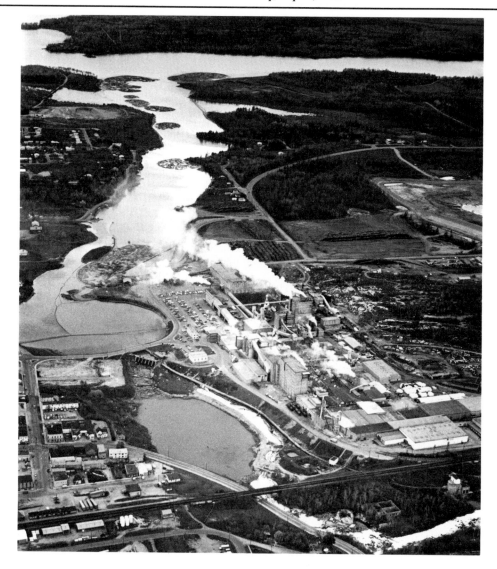

defended the company against southern criticism in fear it might shut down operations. "I like Dryden. I like Reed," sports shop operator Len Barrett would tell reporter Ross Howard of the *Toronto Star*. "This is a one-industry town and the industry feeds us. Those agitators in the south don't live here. I'm bloody sick and tired of the mercury and Indian situation." A clerk in Barrett's store remarked: "Clean it up? I only see it for half a second when I drive over the bridge. Prove to me that the pollution really affects the livelihood of the people downstream."

Before returning to Japan, the Minamata Disease patients joined Indian leaders in a march on the Ontario Legislature at Queen's Park in Toronto. It was a raucous demonstration. Played out before the eyes of the Toronto news media, the mercury issue was revived, after simmering and sputtering for five years.

The publicity which followed the Indians' visit to Minamata, and the return visits by the scientists and patients from Japan, was embarrassing to the provincial and federal governments. Under the spotlight of public attention, they became more receptive to Indian demands for action to correct the medical and economic inequities at Grassy Narrows and Whitedog.

Bill Fobister, who succeeded Andy Keewatin as chief at Grassy in September 1975, said a critical problem facing the band was the pervasive influence of regular monthly welfare cheques on the lives of the people.

"The people would sooner have an exchange of welfare cheques for work," he said. "They would sooner earn their welfare. Welfare has spoiled them. They have sort of lost their initiative to work. But the people are starting to realize that it is not doing them any good."

The "work for welfare" concept was not an original one, but it was difficult to implement. The federal government was not anxious to undermine its nation-wide welfare program by introducing a "workfare" scheme. Welfare was not meant to provide jobs and such a plan could create enormous bureaucratic problems if the same demands were made elsewhere.

"This welfare thing is a real obstacle," Peter Newberry pointed out. "It is terribly important to beat it, and all the thinking Indian people have the same view."

The band thought that money going toward welfare payments should be subsidized to provide a minimum hourly wage which would finance community work projects such as road maintenance, housing construction, garbage disposal and sawmill operation.

Stu Martin, an Indian Affairs representative in Kenora, said the federal policy was unfortunate. He was an avid supporter of the work for welfare idea, having experimented with it himself while working with Indians near Sioux Lookout, about fifty miles northeast of Dryden, where the native people had been turning to alcohol after disease destroyed the beaver population and trapping was closed for five years. The chief there proposed to Martin that his people be paid welfare cheques only if they worked to build a road from Kassabanaka to Big Trout Lake. The road would reduce air freight costs, and building it would give the band something to do.

It was against regulations, but Martin turned a blind eye as teams of Indians began hacking down trees and smoothing the road. An eight-member committee of band members administered the plan, apportioning out welfare vouchers to the workers. In two months the road was rough, but passable. But Ottawa found out about it and forbade further work.

The Indians' distress over the mounting dependence on welfare at Grassy Narrows and Whitedog prompted a meeting, in October 1975, between Indian Affairs Minister Judd Buchanan and the chiefs of the two reserves. They agreed to pool financial allocations from federal and provincial sources, including welfare payments, in an effort to develop a new economic base in the communities.

Under the agreement, the band councils were given assistance by federal officers to draft an annual work plan. It could feature one or two major projects, or several smaller ones, but would provide jobs at minimum wages. Logging operations and community improvement jobs were planned. The federal government agreed to spend $920,000 to fund 125 jobs at the two reserves, $480,000 at Grassy. Meanwhile, the provincial government had budgeted about $1.5 million for capital works and job stimulation, including constuction of the long-promised walk-in freezer to hold fish brought in by truck from Winnipeg.

Once again, there were complications. Due to the already high mercury levels found in the people of Grassy, health authorities set a maximum allowable mercury intake of .2 parts per million in a reduced fish diet, far below the existing federal standard for other populations. Queen's Park had trouble finding a sufficient supply of preferred species which met the tougher standards, and Premier William Davis said the freezer plan would have to be reassessed.

"The provision of fish is not employment-generating," he said. "If the Indians were to grow their own protein, not only would an alternative food supply be available, but employment opportunities would also be provided." The Indians were asked to consider starting a market garden as a pilot project.

Work was launched on a day care center, a service which the authorities hoped would lend some stability to the turbulent lives of youngsters at Grassy. Queen's Park also earmarked funds to provide a community consultant and business advisory services. Davis would later describe the initiatives as "evidence we are not indifferent to the situation."

One of the more promising projects was a federally funded manufacturing enterprise in which a half dozen men were trained to produce fiberglass canoes. The men had to master the knack of operating electrical power tools, but with practice began turning out brightly painted canoes which sold well. Instructor Ruth Vlchek of Red Deer, Alberta, said she was optimistic the project would become a money-making, job-producing venture. "I know they can do a good job, because I've seen them do a good job," she said. "I just hope they have the initiative to keep it going. You can't push these people."

The band council and officials of the federal Indian Affairs department also opened negotiations with a white businessman to build a shoe manufacturing plant on the reserve, but as discussions dragged on, it appeared unlikely the factory would be built.

"The task of generating jobs, making new businesses, well, nine out of ten fail in the city," said Peter Newberry, "so to succeed out here is going to be even tougher."

The make-work schemes reduced unemployment to about 50 per cent. The incidence of drunkenness and violence declined, but remained a lingering problem and Indian leaders debated the merits of holding a referendum to decide whether alcoholic beverages should be allowed on the reserve, where they might be better controlled.

The infusion of provincial and federal funds did little to convince the people that politicians finally had a grip on the problem, only that they were responding to public pressure. Sport fishing in the chain remained an issue. So long as angling was allowed by Queen's Park, and camps continued to operate, the Indians could not expect to be treated as anything but pawns in a game of politics which favored the industry that had disrupted their lives. In December 1975, chiefs and councillors of Grassy Narrows and Whitedog threatened to begin regular deliveries of poisoned fish to the homes of Premier Davis, the leaders of the two Opposition parties in

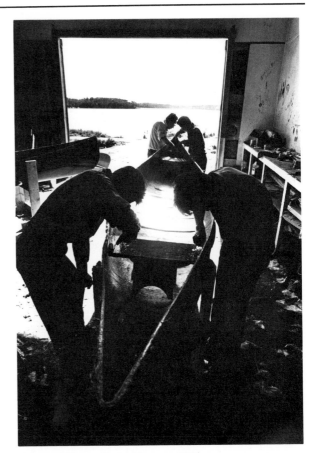

Canoe-making at Grassy Narrows, 1976.

For five years,
we have fought the bias, indifference and hostility
of your minister of natural resources....
It is long enough.

the Ontario Legislature, Health Minister Frank Miller, Attorney-General Roy McMurtry, Natural Resources Minister Bernier and Robert Billingsley, president of Reed.

"We will expect you to share with us the risk to your families and children," the Indians wrote to Davis. "We will expect, sir, that each and every day you will all cause these fish to be suitably prepared and to be eaten in your homes, as they are in ours.

"We feel that continuing consumption of these mercury polluted fish by the children of our political masters will be solid evidence that policy in Ontario does not differentiate between our children and yours — that you, like many of our people, will watch your children eating the poisoned pickerel fillets from these waters, will wonder what is causing personality change, will ask yourself what is the reason for the deterioration in their physical and mental health.

The Indians claimed their people continued to eat poisoned fish because the river system was open to visiting anglers and "the existing policy is nothing more than administration by your government of the death and degradation of our people."

"Legally closing the rivers would do two things," they stated. "It would mean that it was contrary to the law to take fish. Laws can be enforced, but first they must be passed. It would also mean that there would no longer be people taking money from tourists — people who have a direct financial interest in denying that mercury-infected fish are poisonous.

"Fishing camp operators on the polluted rivers

now deny that the fish are poisonous and they effectively require that our people, when guiding guests, cook these poisoned fish, feed them to uninformed and unsuspecting guests and, themselves, eat them. The guides are on the rivers everyday and they poison themselves with these fish everyday.

"They don't fall down dead. So, many Indian people, copying the statements of your minister of natural resources, say: 'See. The fish aren't poisonous' . . .

"We know that the fish are poisonous. We know that eating the fish can destroy the mind and health and take the life of Indians and whites. This cannot fail to be known by anybody who, for five long years, has watched the growing violence, the deteriorating health and the declining morale of our people. . . .

"Unless you act to close these polluted rivers, our people are doomed."

The letter took six pages to convey its message of frustration and resentment against Queen's Park and, specifically, against Leo Bernier.

"For five years, we have fought the bias, indifference and hostility of your minister of natural resources. For five years we have observed the deterioration of the health and morale of our people, have seen violence grow, have lost friends and relations in violent deaths.

"It is long enough. Enough people have died. Enough of our people have been destroyed. Enough lack of understanding. Enough pro-polluter bias. Enough indifference —"

To this and other criticisms of his way of con-

Nearly six years after the initial discovery of mercury in Canadian water, the government was finally sending scientists to countries which had lost hundreds of people to the deadly chemical.

ducting the public's business, Bernier would simply retort, "You can't satisfy everyone."

Bernier was a special kind of cabinet minister: a northerner who felt his part of the province was mistreated and misunderstood by the south, a thick-skinned politician who seemed to disdain his critics. He would take their barbs, and smile. He would use his ministerial influence to take his daughter's father-in-law fishing on a protected lake, then explain he had done nothing illegal. He flatly stated that he had used his influence to have confiscated guns returned to persons convicted under the Game and Fish Act. He explained that he felt the con-fiscatory powers of the act were too great. When game wardens seized two fish left by his daughter's father-in-law to be stuffed and mounted, Bernier had them returned.

Davis refused to close the waterway, at least right away. The matter was under study. A month earlier, the premier had appointed another task force, a team organized by the Ontario ministry of health. During November and December it travelled to Minamata and Iraq to gather on-site information about mercury poison. Nearly six years after the initial discovery of mercury in Canadian waters, government was finally sending scientists to countries which had lost hundreds of people to the deadly chemical.

On its return to Canada, the team told the Davis government what had been obvious to the Indians for years: "Fish from the Wabigoon and lower English River system should not be used for human or animal food. . . . The most effective

method of achieving [this] is to close the waterway to all forms of fishing."

"In particular," the study group reported, "this would protect the fishing guides, who are the popu-lation most at risk." The group said no illnesses had been found which might be directly linked to mer-cury poisoning, but recommended the river closing as a precaution against an outbreak of Minamata Disease, which Japanese observers were beginning to forecast.

The government considered the recommenda-tions, and chose not to act, at least not right away. Davis reaffirmed the government's policy against compensating victims of pollution ("and I do not anticipate any change"), and used the "con-tradictory" medical evidence as cause for further study.

"Medical examination of some residents with the highest levels of mercury in blood and hair has not revealed any symptoms which could not be accounted for by other illnesses or which could be attributed solely to mercury poisoning," he said. "I am aware, of course, that physicians from Japan have said that there are cases of mercury poisoning in the group, but this has not been confirmed either by our own consultants or by non-governmental Canadian medical specialists who were asked to check on the Japanese findings."

"This puts us in the difficult position of appear-ing to deny the existence of a disease which has been diagnosed by foreign consultants," the premier acknowledged. "The only way that we can resolve this problem is to do further investigations. There are, in fact, several co-operating groups, both within and outside the government, which are studying the matter. Very soon, there will be a comprehensive investigation of the whole situation, with particular emphasis on the health of the residents."

Six years after the discovery of excessive mercury levels in the bodies of Indians in northwestern Ontario, the premier was promising another "comprehensive" study. Between studies, Tommy Keesick's wife had given birth to their first child. It was a boy. The Keesicks named him Teruo, after Teruo Kawamoto, who had courageously carried the protests of pollution victims to the gates of industry in Minamata. The fear Keesick had expressed in Japan that young Teruo might be born with Minamata Disease proved unfounded. Unlike other babies from Grassy Narrows born lifeless or sickly, Teruo Keesick gave no signs that he might be suffering from mercury poisoning.

10
The Shadows that Remained

"Do you think Keith has Minamata Disease, Marcel?"

Marcel Pahpasay hesitated. His four-year-old son bounced on the bed beside him, crying incomprehensibly. "I'm pretty sure," the father said finally. "Yes, I'm pretty sure he has."

There was no sense of conviction in his answer. Medical experts were at a loss to confirm or deny that Keith's deformed arms and legs and apparent mental retardation had been caused by mercury in the fish eaten by his mother Rosy as she carried her son inside her. However, the Pahpasays had seen a film brought back from Minamata and in the misshapen Japanese children, innocent victims of congenital mercury poisoning, the Indian parents saw Keith, his sightless eyes wandering, his limbs beginning to contort.

"That's what mercury poisoning looks like," said Dr. Peter Newberry in a 1976 television interview. The camera showed Keith's deformities and this image plus Newberry's statement set off a controversy regarding the cause of the child's affliction.

Keith was born six weeks prematurely in hospital in Kenora, and three times stopped breathing. Oxygen loss could have caused brain damage. That could be the explanation for the cerebral palsy that doomed Keith to live out his life under constant care in the handicapped children's unit of a Thunder Bay hospital. The Pahpasays can seldom visit their son. He is too far from home.

As a guide, Marcel Pahpasay consumed a steady diet of fish. So did Rosy, who often joined her husband on his trips away from Grassy Narrows. What

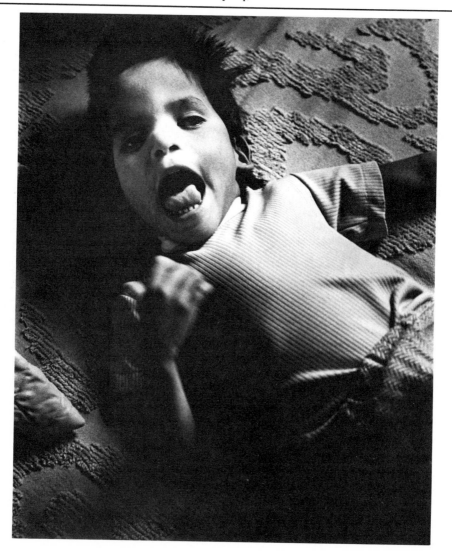

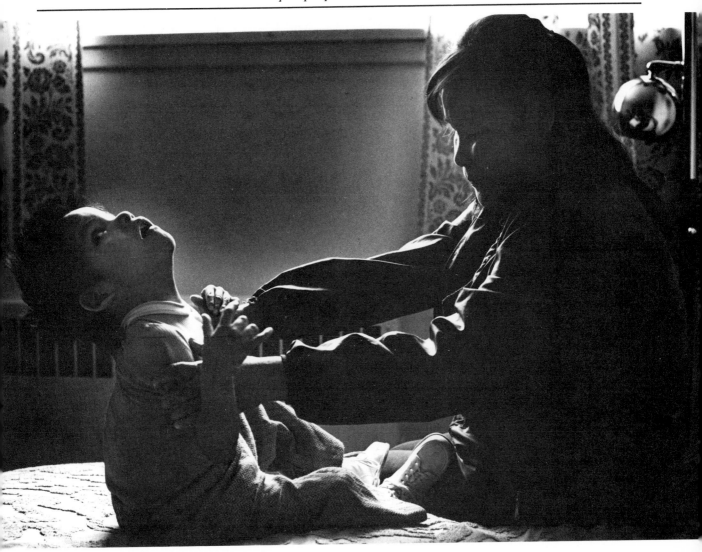

they saw on the film, the tragedy of children whose lives were destroyed before they began, made them suspect that their baby had been struck by the same poison.

But no one could be sure. James Walker, administrator of Thunder Bay's Walter Hogarth Memorial Hospital, said: "It is impossible to determine why the boy was born that way. We just don't know." Dr. Peter Neelands, Keith's attending physician, also said it would be very difficult to determine what had caused the boy's condition. On the basis of mercury tests conducted three years after the child's birth, Dr. Bette Stephenson, then acting minister of health for Ontario, said she suspected the boy did not have mercury poisoning and "no responsible physician" would make a definite diagnosis. In fact, only an autopsy could reveal the amount of mercury in the Pahpasay child's organs. Once again, the people of Grassy Narrows could only guess whether mercury had damaged their lives.

Keith bounced on the bed, arching his back and dropping, each time emitting a little shriek, somehow communicating his happiness with his parents' visit. Marcel looked down at his son and smiled.

"He has never spoken, but he makes noises. He was a normal baby. We didn't notice anything wrong until he was a year old. Then he got sick. Every time he had a cold, he really had a hard time. So we had to take him to the hospital. That's when we found out he was blind.

"His arms and legs weren't like that before. His hands and feet are just starting to go like that."

Marcel said he was worried by his family's experiences: his own high mercury levels, those of his wife, the stillbirth of the earlier child, Keith's incurable brain damage and the feisty temperament of another son, Clark.

"Clark has high mercury levels," the father commented, "and he's the kind of guy who has a bad temper. You can't control him, and he's only about six or seven. I quit guiding about three summers ago when I noticed about my kids. Now all I do is work around the reserve."

Keith bounced again and squealed, gripping Marcel's finger as his hand came near.

"That's the way he does all the time. When you talk to him he listens, and when you leave him alone he starts jumping again. He will always be in the hospital. That's what they told me. He has a bad spine. But the way his feet are turning. His wrists. His hands. He used to see a little bit, I think, but he can't see anymore."

Marcel wanted answers, but none was available.

"Can they find out how much mercury there is in a baby who dies?" he asked.

"You mean your baby? The one buried at Jones?"

"Yes."

"I don't think so. It's too late now."

"Oh."

Reports of the many tragedies in the lives of the Grassy Narrows Indians had been printed and broadcast for six years before whites organized in support of the natives' cause. In February of 1976, a white group mounted a protest against Reed Paper.

The company had sponsored an art display entitled "Changing Visions — Canadian Landscape," a collection of paintings of outdoor scenes. About two hundred and fifty demonstrators turned out when the touring display opened at the Art Gallery of Ontario in Toronto. They hoped to convince other whites that Reed's public relations gesture was hypocritical and should be boycotted.

"Join the line! Don't go in!" the pickets shouted, sometimes jostling and hissing at gallery visitors who refused to be turned back by the demonstration. Those who entered the show were offered pieces of frozen fish. "One of the girls with us was elbowed and verbally attacked," complained one young woman. An organizer of the protest reminded the crowd, "It's not the patrons who are the villains."

The increasingly bad publicity continued to irritate residents of Kenora and Dryden, who feared a devastating loss in tourist income if the "attacks" in the southern media persisted.

"Gutter journalism is not new," the *Dryden Observer* snapped. "As with fashions in clothing, it seems to poke its ugly nose above the muck with cynical regularity . . . . There are some journalists who seem to derive a perverse delight from upsetting, disturbing and hurting people. They are the products of our Canadian star system for journalists, taught to make noise rather than sense. And quite often, the coverage these people give to an issue appears more designed to stroke their exaggerated egos than to inform the public or to convey a truth."

Politically the fires were being stoked, and Health Minister Frank Miller confessed "I've come closer to quitting politics over this issue than anything else." Miller and his cabinet colleagues, however, did not follow the advice of their own health team to close down the polluted waterways. The health minister said: "I don't think closing the river to sport fishing would save one Indian."

The dilemma begged and defied solution. In Ottawa and Toronto, politicians considered the possibility of closing the waterway to fishing and expropriating camp property as steps toward converting the region into a wilderness park for the century it would remain polluted. The Indians were told they could count on government funding if they wanted to take the polluter to court. The suggestion was even made that the villages of Grassy Narrows and Whitedog might be moved to uncontaminated areas.

"We've already moved from one spot to here," Andy Keewatin remarked. "How many times do they want us to move?"

The Indians had never asked to be relocated. Roy McDonald, one of the Indian leaders from Whitedog, said violence might erupt if the government did not start paying attention to what the Indians *were* saying. The growing tension was like the wind coming from the west side of the lake, he remarked. "When it starts it is nothing. But by the time it gets to the east side it has built up. That's what it is like. It is building up, and it is not of our making.

"Before, we were not political, except the chief

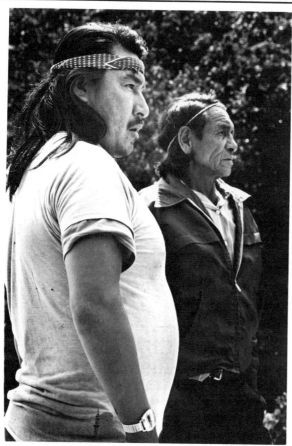

No trespassing, Whitedog, 1976.

and maybe one or two others. We were homey and comfortable. But the younger ones now, well, their feelings are building up like the wind."

As summer once again arrived in English River country, so did Teruo Kawamoto, the angry young man of Minamata, come to Canada to speak about mercury pollution. He visited the Indians and did not hide his concern over their failure to move the government to positive action.

"To my regret," he said in June 1976, "the awareness of the people has not progressed as much as I would have liked. The life style of these people was primitive and the environmental impact was enormous. The modernization, the technology and all the changes they have had to face have had an effect, their lack of awareness of what has been happening."

Unlike the militancy of Minamata, which was always stormy, sometimes violent, the protests by the Canadian Indians were generally undramatic and attracted only superficial press attention and public interest. One of the reasons was the backlash among conservative native people over the Anicinabe Park occupation, a contentious confrontation that lost the Indians as many friends as it gained.

But the situation demanded some form of action and that June militancy again surfaced as a means of getting a message across to government. Residents of Whitedog, after much debate and soul searching, decided to block a road through their reserve which provided sportsmen access to four tourist camps north of Whitedog. "Let us commercial fish or close

Chief Isaac Mandamin, Whitedog roadblock, 1976.

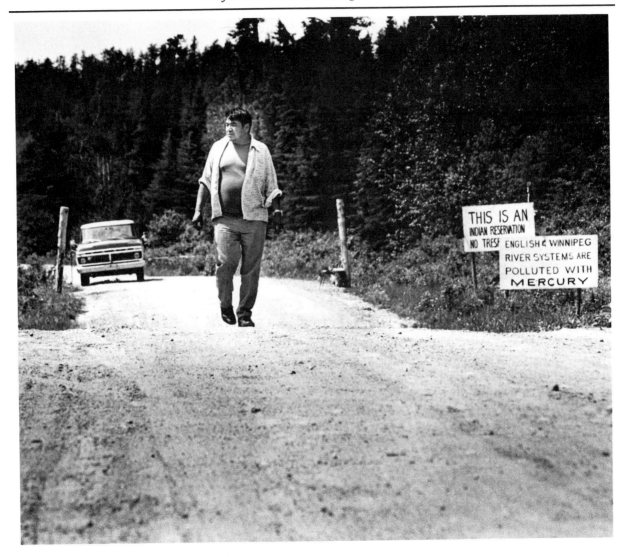

THIS IS AN
INDIAN RESERVATION
NO TRESP ENGLISH & WINNIPEG
RIVER SYSTEMS ARE
POLLUTED WITH
MERCURY

down sports fishing," said Isaac Mandamin, the chief. "Let's find out for sure if mercury is here."

The Indians erected a blockade and posted signs: "This road is closed due to health hazards." "This checkpoint is peaceful and lawful." The demonstration was ineffectual. Anglers deterred by the roadblock could be flown into the camps.

The federal government felt the establishment of a national park might provide a solution. If the native people agreed with the idea, the camps could be bought by the government and all fishing inside the polluted boundaries forbidden. Three weeks after setting up the blockade, the Indians took it down and agreed to consider the park proposal. But the plan was later scrapped because the Indians concluded it "would not solve their immediate social and economic problems."

The press attention drawn by such demonstrations upset camp operators throughout the district, both on and off polluted waterways. At a meeting held in Ear Falls in the fall of 1976, they blamed the news media for offering the public a distorted view of the problem. Those whose camps were on clean waters complained that their business had dropped 25 per cent or more because the media were not specifying which lakes on the English-Wabigoon chain were the polluted bodies. But one man in the crowd suggested the target of their wrath might be incorrect. "We've been going around for the last five years with our heads in the sand," he said. "Somewhat by design. I'd stand corrected, but I believe the directors of the Northern Ontario Tourist Outfitters Association agreed some five or

six years ago not to talk about mercury to the media. We kinda hoped it would go away."

At Grassy Narrows, another problem remained unsolved. Although unemployment had been slightly reduced by make-work projects, and violence had declined under the continued surveillance of the police, alcohol remained a disruptive influence. Indian leaders, many of them heavy drinkers, decided to allow alcohol to be brought onto the reserve, the rationale being that consumption could be better policed on the reserve than in Kenora. Schoolchildren posted signs opposing the plan, but in a February 1976 referendum in which only 69 out of 138 eligible voters cast ballots, the band voted, 49 to 20, to bring liquor back to their homes. The Indian Affairs department eventually approved the plan and alcohol was allowed onto the reserve in the spring.

"People will have to learn how to manage their drinks," said Bill Fobister. "They'll have to learn how to handle it to keep their jobs."

The mastery of social drinking, however, still eluded the Indians of Grassy: there was an increase in drinking and a return to the ugly family quarrels. One of the OPP commented, "A policeman's dream is to have nothing to do, and we were almost at that point. Now, after two weeks, it is as bad as it was when we first came here."

A drunken Indian who bore the scars of an attack by his wife the previous night asked "Does drinking keep the mercury down?"

"No, it has no effect," he was told. "Is that what the people think, that it keeps it down?"

"Yes, That's what they say."

Attendance at school, always a problem, fell off with the rising incidence of alcohol abuse. The school purchased four bicycles as prizes in a contest to reduce truancy. Draw tickets were awarded every two weeks — three tickets for perfect attendance, two for missing only a half-day and one if only one day was missed. "Attend school so you can win tickets," a sign pleaded with pupils.

The pressure of trying to help his people recover their sense of self-worth and dignity proved too severe for Bill Fobister, who gave up the position of chief in March 1976, after serving for seven months. He had strained his nerves and lost too much weight, but Fobister agreed to continue as special projects manager.

Fobister was not alone in his feeling of hopelessness and bureaucratic entanglement. Jeff Perkins, a social worker appointed by the Ontario Government in January to co-ordinate federal and provincial programs on the Whitedog and Grassy Narrows reserves, lasted only three months before quitting because of "uncertainties I can't live with." Perkins had been appointed to help the two bands make best use of senior government assistance in their struggle for economic redevelopment. But he soon discovered what the Indians had known for years: action did not flow as smoothly as words from Queen's Park. Perkins said that while the idea of co-ordinating programs was sound, long delays in approving funds often scuttled good intentions.

When Bill Fobister announced his decision to quit as Grassy's chief, no one wanted the job. Three men were nominated to the position, but each dropped out before an election could be held. As ninety-eight eligible voters gathered in the community hall to pick a new leader, there were still no likely successors.

The least obvious choice was, perhaps, Joe Quoquat, a twenty-eight-year-old clerk at the Hudson's Bay store. Quoquat seldom spoke to anyone. However, the people respected his ability to support a wife and three children at a time when most depended wholly on welfare.

The election meeting was awkward. Each person looked into the eyes of others in an uncertain search for leadership. Someone mentioned Quoquat's name and a majority of the audience rose and drifted toward him in a gesture of support. The reluctant chief said, "I'll try my best. I can't make too many promises."

Bill Fobister knew what weight had been shifted to Quoquat's frail shoulders. In recent months he had found himself hitting the bottle with increasing regularity.

"I'm missing work," Fobister confessed. "I didn't come to work yesterday due to a big hangover. The people see us as leaders, and we drink with our people, and they think, 'why should we not drink?' But I have made a verbal agreement with my wife this morning. Now is the time to act. Me, as a leader, I am making a fresh start. I'll stop drinking, even if it takes me a while."

"Being a leader, you've got to be responsible," said the former chief, tears of anguish welling up in his eyes. "You've got to show your people you want

It's really tough being a leader at Grassy. You try to do something for your people and you turn around and it's not worth it.

Bill Fobister

to do the best in a way they will follow. Right now, I think I'm losing the respect of some of the people I drink with. But if they see that I don't drink, maybe they will say 'why don't we stop?'"

Fobister harbored a guilt which contributed to his anxiety. He had promoted the referendum which permitted alcohol to be brought onto the reserve. He watched as the men of the band overindulged, undermining the very work programs he was struggling to establish.

"I feel kinda bad about it," he said, "because I let it go through. Maybe we should have another vote. Things were going well before. Oh man, they were sure going well. We started to get along with the police. But now they have to really crack down. We have to correct this situation.

"People used to say that the people of Grassy don't have a mercury problem. They have an alcohol problem. Now, maybe, it is our number one problem. At the moment I think it is. There are other problems, too, but we've got to solve this drinking problem first, because this is going to ruin us. I really feel bad about it."

"It's really tough being a leader at Grassy," he said. "You try to do something for your people and you turn around and it's not worth it."

"Until the people realize this alcohol thing is their problem, then things won't get better here. I'm responsible to my kids, my family. I'll just have to taper off my drinking. I don't want to lose that. And until the people start to think about that, things won't get better.

"If they keep on like this – kids being neglected and all that – one of these days their kids are going to end up killing themselves, or even starving.

"I don't know how to solve this problem. I think I'll talk to the others about this drinking and see what we can do to make this a good place to live in."

Joe Quoquat was still learning his new job as chief when he faced his first challenge. During a tour of area reserves in May, Stephen Lewis, the leader of the New Democratic party, and accompanying reporters from Toronto were confronted by the stench of about five thousand pounds of fish rotting in the community freezer at Grassy Narrows. Controversy once again hit the southern press.

The fish were part of a ten-thousand-pound shipment of whitefish from Manitoba, arranged by the Ontario government to replace poisoned fish from the English River in the Indians' diet. The freezer had been shut down and the pungent aroma of decaying fish soon filled the air. Who was to blame?

Indian residents said the fish were already turning bad when the shipment arrived, and Quoquat told the reporters that government officials had been notified two weeks earlier that the freezer was not working. At Queen's Park, Natural Resources Minister Bernier wrote off the incident as "sabotage". A police investigation later concluded that youngsters had vandalized the freezer, but Bernier refused to withdraw his charge that it had been sabotaged.

In Toronto, Robert Billingsley, the beleaguered president of Reed Paper, repeated his sense of moral and social responsibility for troubles caused by pol-

**When I sit back objectively and I look and say, what is the problem there . . .
I don't get a very clear picture . . .
The leads must come from governments. . . .**
Robert W. Billingsley

lution, but said his company was obliged to depend upon government for leadership in the search for solutions.

"When I sit back objectively and I look and say, what is the problem there and what could we as a company, or I personally as head of the company, do to help that situation, I don't get a very clear picture," he said.

"I get [the picture of] local Indians with some concern. They've got a problem. But very little clear-cut direction of where they'd like to go and what they'd like to do in terms of making a viable social community out of that, which means they need an economic life and all the other factors that go with a reasonably modern life. . . .

"The leads must come from governments, and I'm not going to say which government, because I think it's very unclear as to who should do what. That's a problem in this country, between federal and provincial jurisdictions, resources and all sorts of things. It's manifest in this case on a small number of people who do not have a very good life style at this point in time.

"I'm not sure they ever had a very good life style, but at least at this point in time I don't see how they are going to get a better life style unless something is done to address the socio-economic life of those communities."

"I don't think we are sociologists," explained Billingsley. "I don't think we have the expertise there. We must rely on others. Where we do have expertise is in the economic life and the business life and I have said the kinds of things where we might be able to help is in setting up the kind of employment opportunities that might be beneficial to people. . . ." Despite its wealth of business knowledge, Reed Paper chose not to send company representatives onto the reserves to offer assistance.

"In terms of compensation, if there is a legal problem, then there should be a legal solution, and we would obviously respond accordingly. What I am talking about is simply from the point of view of being a good social corporate citizen and trying to do something in an area where I think we can be of some help. . . .

"What that role will be will depend on what the government is doing and what the Indians want. I don't think it's our job to say we think you should put a sawmill there and we'll help you build it or donate some things or help you run it or buy the wood from it or supply the wood to it or any kind of thing. Because if the government is going to build a sawmill, then our suggestion doesn't make any sense. Maybe they don't want sawmills. Maybe they'd much prefer to get into a cottage industry type of thing, or maybe wild rice, and they'd like some help in that area."

Reed's position from the day the mercury was discovered was that the company had met all government regulations and therefore could not be held legally accountable for the damage done by the pollutant. "Even Stephen Lewis has made a big point of saying that he has found no evidence that we have broken any laws. This is the tragedy of this whole thing," the company president said.

"Here's a classic case of an industrial society

using a chemical to help make a product we all use, paper. It's not a frivolous thing. We might say we use too much of it. Nevertheless, we can't eliminate paper from the society....

"At that time, we did not have the knowledge that this thing was potentially as dangerous as it turned out to be. I'm confident that there are a number of chemicals in the world today in all sorts of industries which, ten years from now, we will find there is either some real or potential damage. My concern is, how is society going to deal with this kind of situation? It's a problem for society.

"It's easy to say, 'Let the polluter pay.' I think, as a principle, that makes sense. When you have defined rules for pollution and you say, 'Do anything other than that, then you are wrong and you pay.' But we weren't breaking any rules...."

If Billingsley was at a loss for solutions, he was not alone. The crisis posed a political conundrum for Premier Davis of Ontario and Judd Buchanan, one of three ministers of Indian Affairs who had watched the situation deteriorate.

"The situation is highly complex with many, many facets to it," the premier stressed. "It will take a great deal of time and effort as well as money to resolve. We are committed to resolving it in the best interests of the native people and therefore are involving them in our attempts to find the solutions. Results are being achieved," he said, "albeit, not as quickly as we would wish, but given the complexity of the situation we are making progress and we hope the rate of progress will be accelerated...."

"We are all agreed that the whole matter is a most unfortunate, most perplexing and most challenging problem and one which must be resolved in the best interests not only of the people now living in the area, but of future generations of Ontarians. It will take the combined efforts and energies of a good many people, both in and out of government, working together in a spirit of mutual respect and co-operation, to arrive at practicable and humanitarian solutions."

His response was not unlike that of Buchanan, the federal minister responsible for administration of the contentious Indian Act, which charged Ottawa with the dubious responsibility to oversee and protect Canada's native peoples. Buchanan, a former insurance man from London, Ontario, was Indian Affairs Minister from August of 1974 until October of 1976, and was often under fire from dissatisfied Indian leaders. Some called for his resignation.

"I'd be misleading you if I suggested I enjoy being kicked at," Buchanan once said. "Regular calls for my resignation. This sort of thing. But I accept that this is, to a degree, part of the process of finding a way....

"They say I interfere too much. I agree with that. There is nothing that would delight me more than to 'shove off' on the Indian people more responsibility for their own affairs. But then they say I just want to get rid of them and shuck off my job. Then they say I'm interfering. I am an impediment to them. It's a difficult row to hoe."

Buchanan said the problems confronting the people of Grassy Narrows and Whitedog had challenged the efforts of six federal departments and agencies and had used up a flood of investment capital in a vain attempt to put things right.

"The situation has indeed had a tragic effect on the two reserves," he said. "It is all the more unfortunate when it is realized that, despite any efforts or processes now known it will be many years before the river system will be cleansed of the mercury. . . ."

Buchanan said his department's files on the initial decision to relocate the village of Grassy Narrows to its new site were "unfortunately very sketchy." He acknowledged that the relocation had had a profound social impact "but, with the river pollution being so closely tied in with their lives, it is difficult to determine the extent of the hardships imposed."

He said the federal government's policy for years has been against encouraging relocation without the consent of the band. "If relocation is an issue, we will assist bands financially for the purposes of research and other activities necessary to ensure adequate compensation. We do not encourage Indian people living in isolated communities to relocate in more urban areas but, through our education program, we try to provide the Indian people with an option of remaining in a community, or moving.

"Certainly, the clash between any isolated community, including Grassy Narrows, and an industrialized non-Indian community can result in very serious problems. . . . We give the people the opportunity of making a choice on the kind of life they wish to follow. If Indian people such as those at Grassy Narrows choose to remain on the reserve, we try as much as possible to assist them in meeting their needs in education, employment and their preferred way of life."

By 1976, the news media had inundated the public with stories about the mercury crisis. The mere mention of mercury conjured up images of dead Indians and the Reed Paper Company. It was impossible to imagine the company's public image becoming more controversial. Then, Cree and Ojibway Indians in the region of Treaty Nine, in the far northwest corner of the province, discovered the extent of Reed's interest in the province's black spruce forest.

The black spruce is one of the most widely distributed trees in Canada, found in each of the ten provinces and in some parts of the Northwest Territories. It is a vigorous species, but in northern climes grows slowly. Reed, in collaboration with Leo Bernier's ministry of natural resources, proposed exploitation of 18,983 square miles of the untouched forest, home to about two thousand native people. Other Indians in the region trapped within the proposed timber tract, which extended roughly three hundred miles east from the Ontario-Manitoba border.

Reed and the government, the Indians learned, were discussing methods of establishing a giant pulp and paper mill in the Red Lake-Ear Falls area, a $400-million installation which would process a thousand tons of wood daily and provide about twelve hundred jobs.

In June, Chief Andrew Rickard, president of

**Rickard said on the basis of past experience,
asking the Indians to trust the government was like
"asking Colonel Sanders to babysit our chickens."**

Grand Council, Treaty Nine, travelled to Toronto, where he held a press conference and tore up a photocopy of the treaty, claiming violation of the 1905 agreement. He said the Indians would die before allowing Reed to ruin their homeland as it had done to lands owned by the people of Grassy Narrows and Whitedog.

"It's a sell-out of the first order," said Rickard, "which will hurt not just my people, but all of Ontario. When Reed's greed has destroyed that forest, there will be no wilderness and eventually no timber for anyone."

The northern chief claimed his ancestors had greeted the white man with trust and open arms, and had helped him to survive the harsh environment, only to see it despoiled.

"Look about you today," Rickard said. "Are white people not ashamed? Do they not have human compassion? Do they not realize that they have literally destroyed everything we've had? All we have is our lives! Now they want that, too, through greed that perpetuates cultural genocide.

"Can you not see what has happened? Visitors were welcomed to a paradise. But within three hundred years they've turned it into a living hell and a garbage dump. They've destroyed and destroyed, until there is little left to destroy.

"And now white eyes look to the last frontier — as they call it — and plan to destroy the only part of the land left in a natural state as created by the Great Spirit. But if it should die, my people will die. I will too! And this shall come to all, since death does not discriminate.

"Hear what I am saying. Indeed, it could well be the key to your survival too. . . . Today it stops. We will not tolerate this suppression and destruction any longer. Our children and future generations will be protected at any cost."

J. K. Reynolds, a deputy minister in Bernier's ministry, insisted that no agreement had been reached with Reed and he promised that if an agreement was concluded, it would provide for a full public inquiry to guarantee that social and environmental concerns were met.

"But I don't blame the Indians for being apprehensive," he said. "History and modern technology have not been kind to them."

The Indians, however, were much more than apprehensive. They were outraged, and they launched a publicity campaign to force a royal commission of inquiry into the whole question of northern development and resource exploitation. Reed and the government insisted that the new project would be environmentally sound, but the Indians would not believe them.

Rickard said on the basis of past experience, asking the Indians to trust the government was like "asking Colonel Sanders to babysit our chickens."

Billingsley of Reed said the Indians' distrust of government was a "tragic situation." "There's no question that they are against us. There could be many reasons for that. I think, though, the government, which is the law of the land, must be the final authority. There is no other, except anarchy. And therefore, I think it is a matter of government working with the Indians to try to convince them that they are going to have a fair hearing."

If the experiences of the people of Grassy Narrows and Whitedog were insufficient cause for distrust, the provincial government's record on forest management was more than sufficient. The government had assumed the responsibility for regeneration programs in 1962, but less than a half of cut areas were being reforested.

K. W. Hearnden, chairman of the school of forestry at Lakehead University in Thunder Bay, told a northern forest symposium there was nothing to suggest the trend would be reversed.

"It is my belief," he said, "that in all probability Canadian forest history will reflect faithfully that of other countries. The mostly unregulated, uncontrolled, mechanized assault upon our northern forests, governed only by the consideration of minimum current wood extraction cost, will continue. The conversion of our northern forests to hard currency, with a minimal commitment of effort to the establishment of a high-quality second forest for the benefit of future generations, must be anticipated."

An environmental planner inside Bernier's ministry warned in an internal memo that failure to achieve a better regenerative rate "will likely lead to a timber shortage by the year 2000."

On October 26, 1976, Bernier announced that he and Billingsley had that day signed a memorandum of understanding to study the feasibility of a mill. The government agreed to conduct an inventory of trees in the tract, taking as long as eighteen months, while the company would conduct an environmental impact study and post a $500,000 bond to fulfill its obligations if a licence was subsequently granted. Bernier said public hearings would be held under the Environmental Assessment Act to ensure an environmentally sound operation.

Rickard dismissed the memorandum as "a death warrant for our people. Through this agreement we have been told that we are to die. The destruction of our environment is our destruction too."

The chief later wrote to the premier, vowing that the Crees and Ojibways would fight the development, to the death if necessary.

"Do not misunderstand us, as some of your ministers seem to do," he wrote. "The campaign to stop the Reed expansion is not another example of southern manipulation of the north. This fight is being waged by a nation of people who have inhabited northern Ontario for thousands of years. It is we who face destruction. It is we who determine our stand. We welcome the support of all people — northerners and southerners alike — but it is the Cree-Ojibway people who lead this struggle . . . .

"We cannot afford to gamble with the lives of children yet unborn. This monstrous project must not be implemented. We are determined to protect our lives and environment at all cost. If you were put in the position that your government has put us in, your reaction would be the same. If we take a passive stand on this major issue, we will dishonor our ancestors and disinherit our children."

Barney Lamm, who himself had a $3.7 million legal claim against Reed Paper, argued that the government should freeze the company's development plans until it had compensated the Indians and camp operators affected by mercury from the Dryden mill. "The solution," he said, "is for the government to tell Reed Paper to clean up its mess and take care of the people who have been hurt." Although this course of action would benefit Lamm, the simple logic of the proposal had merit. The government, however, had demonstrated its weakness in dealing with large companies to achieve environmental improvements. In the case of compensation, it had had no luck at all. If "getting tough" was the suggested answer, one had to look no farther than Dow Chemical to realize that the government was unwilling to seriously chance the economic viability of an industry over environmental matters. The multi-million-dollar legal action against Dow was entering its seventh year, hopelessly enmeshed in a web of claims and counter-claims, with no resolution in sight.

Dow's defence rested almost totally on the argument that it had met all existing governmental regulations at its Sarnia plant, and therefore could not be held accountable for damages from some unpredictable phenomenon.

"At all times [Dow] ... acted within the normal bounds of current and general engineering and scientific knowledge," argued the company's statement of defence, "and within the bounds of good and accepted industrial hygiene practice and in good faith and, further, that upon being advised of the possibility of harm resulting from mercury, it acted expeditiously and properly and under the authority and with the expressed knowledge and permission of the OWRC."

Like the Indians of the north, the fishermen of Lake St. Clair sought recompense for their years of suffering, but as fishing seasons passed, the lake spotted only by anglers, they grew more and more resigned to a working life on land, tending farm crops, pumping gas or enduring the boredom of a factory assembly line. There was cause for bitterness, but little hope for justice.

"That young man — Fimreite, I think it was," grumbled Lawrence Drouillard about Norvald Fimreite, the scientist who had discovered the mercury in Lake St. Clair, "I think if he had kept his nose out of our business we'd still be fishing. Nobody would have got sick anyway. They blew it all out of proportion. They blew it up to an extent they couldn't stop it. And who suffered by it? The little commercial fisherman of Lake St. Clair! We were the only ones to suffer."

It seemed that way to Pat Hamilton also. He could look out his front door and see the anglers enjoying themselves on Lake St. Clair, and it bothered him; his $1,900 pound net boat sold for $300, his fishing equipment in mothballs, his wife working to put food on the table, both of them pushing forty.

"I've been trying to get onto the other lakes to fish, but there doesn't seem to be many opportunities," said Hamilton, who had seen the years pass at odd jobs. "Without an education you don't stand much of a chance nowadays."

The pollution, he said, "wasted the best five years of my life. We was just getting things going, where we were making a good living, then they put us out of business. When you take away five years

Marion Lamm returns to Ball Lake, 1976.

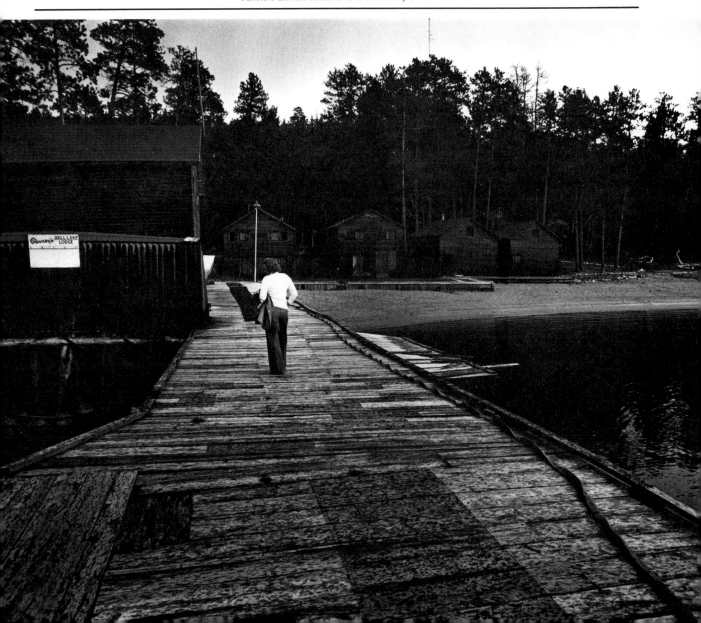

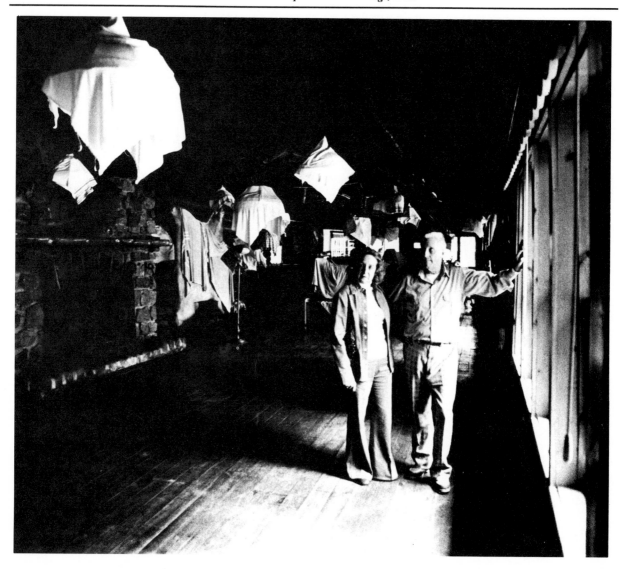

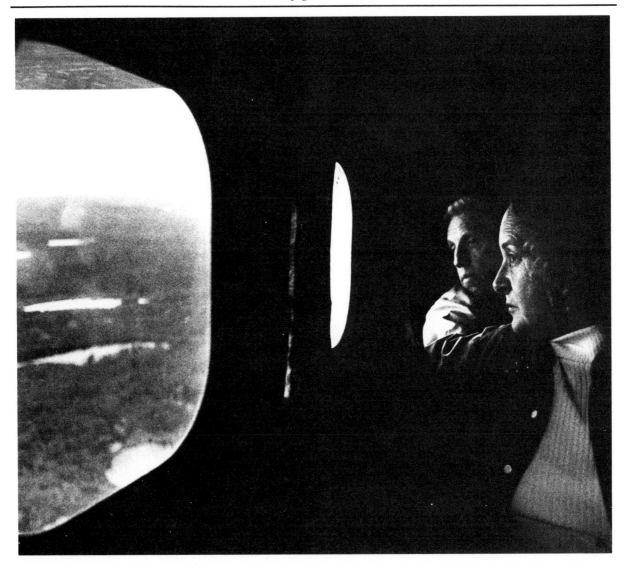

when you're my age, it means a lot. You want to build a little nest egg, but it gets harder every year."

In shoreline warehouses around Lake St. Clair, the fishing nets were rotting. In the north, too, there were sad signs of vanished better times.

Joe Loon was on the dock when the Lamms arrived on an inspection visit of the lodge at Ball Lake. The camp seemed suspended in time, as if the guests had just packed up and left minutes ago. Joe Loon was the last Indian employee at the lodge; he spent the summers acting as caretaker.

Marion Lamm slipped into the chapel and sat for a while in a quiet pew. "These windows came from the church I went to when I was a little girl," she said. "We bought them when they built a new church. I bought them for fifty dollars apiece and we went down in a truck and brought them up. We put them in between old mattresses and trucked them up. They're real old."

They walked into the recreation hall where dances had been held. The firetruck sat, dusty, in a corner. "Used to have a lot of good fun here every Saturday night, eh, Joe?" Marion remarked.

"Yeah," said the Indian, "but no more Saturday nights. I just go to bed."

In the main lodge, sheets covered everything. The Tiffany lamps hung in shadows and, here and there, there were empty spaces on the log walls. Only a shadow of the lodge's former elegance still remained.

"Joe, where's the picture?" Barney asked.

"That's lost," Joe Loon replied.

"It was here last year."

"Yeah, when I got here in the spring, it was gone. Last fall it was here when I left. Somebody's used the fireplace too. They used cabin five."

"There's a knife missing from that wall too," Barney noticed. "They took the horn too. The horn's gone too. Little things. . . . They're not worth a hundred dollars, but it annoys the hell out of me."

"Indians, Joe?" Marion asked.

"Nope. White men. American beer cans."

Barney walked the path outside, scanning with a frown the lodge and cabins, his former home and the outdoor play house where his daughters had spent summer afternoons.

"You know what I've given thought to, real serious thought. Come in here with a bucket of gas and go to every . . . building and throw it in and burn it up."

"Why would you do that?"

"Well, we would have the satisfaction that at least [someone] didn't steal it, or take it away from us."

The visit to Ball Lake was brief, but it rekindled the Lamm's determination to see through the campaign they had started six years earlier.

"We're going to fight it through and we are going to win it, and we're going to get some satisfaction out of winning it," stated Barney. "Every time that we can uncover or bring something to light that embarrasses Bernier or the government, I get enjoyment. We feel that we are right and have been right all along."

Marion Lamm said: "Sooner or later they are going to have to answer to the Lamms — Barney or me or one of the children. . . ."

Meanwhile, at Grassy, the people continued to struggle against their social problems. Piles of beer cases and empty liquor and wine bottles grew high on the stoops of houses, visual evidence, if any more were needed, of the deteriorating morale within the community.

During one November weekend drinking bout, a shotgun blast was heard and another statistic recorded. The Fobister family had lost another member. This time it was David, the band's young social counsellor. Police arrested and laid a charge of non-capital murder against Joe Quoquat, chief of Grassy Narrows.

The people of Grassy Narrows were still in mourning when they picked a new chief, David's twenty-year-old brother Simon.

Simon had lost parents, a grandparent, cousins and now a brother in alcohol-related deaths, and he pledged himself to try to stop the violence that was consuming his people. He proposed that drunks be blacklisted from jobs provided by the band and suggested another referendum might be needed to banish alcohol from the reserve.

11

Returning to the Old Village

The swallows flitted through the open windows of the old council house as Gabe Kokohopenace cut up potatoes for planting, with hands callused from casting nets and setting traps. The rakes, hoes and shovels that leaned against the scarred log walls were symbols of the middle-aged man's new life style, that of a market gardener, working a small plot of cultivated land at the old village where Grassy had its roots, temporarily forgotten though they might be.

"I used to live at the new village," he said. "But my house burned down a couple years ago. Now I work the trap line and spend the summer in an old cabin here."

Partially, at least, he had recaptured the past. Its pleasant memories were still vivid for him, recollections of the days before the old village was abandoned.

"My problem's my kids, you know," said Gabe. "I don't like them getting into mischief. I see a lot of kids over there [at the new village] getting sick. There's too much going on — night life and things like that. Sniffing gas. My kids, now, they turn in at eight-thirty or nine o'clock and they are ready to go in the morning. That's the kind of life I like to see for them. Someday, I guess, I'll return to my tribe, but I'm kind of a selfish guy.

"I have two big boys and I'm teaching them how to trap. They're not amateurs. They're getting pretty good at it. We like it this way."

Gabe remembered how his children began drifting into problems after mercury was discovered and the adults hit the bottle. He tried to keep busy on

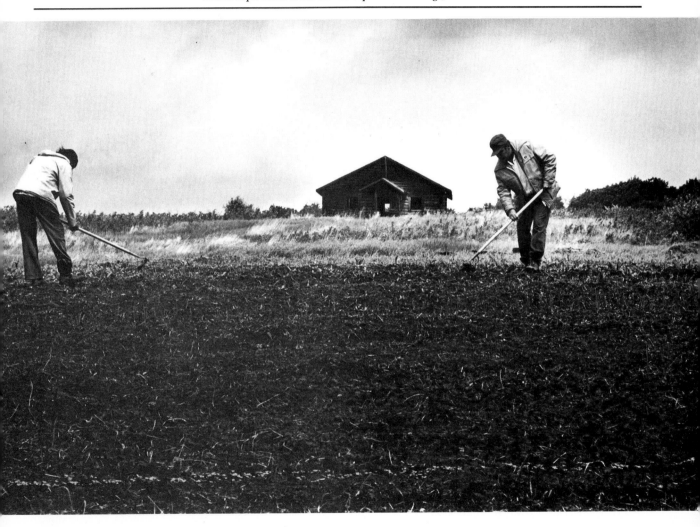

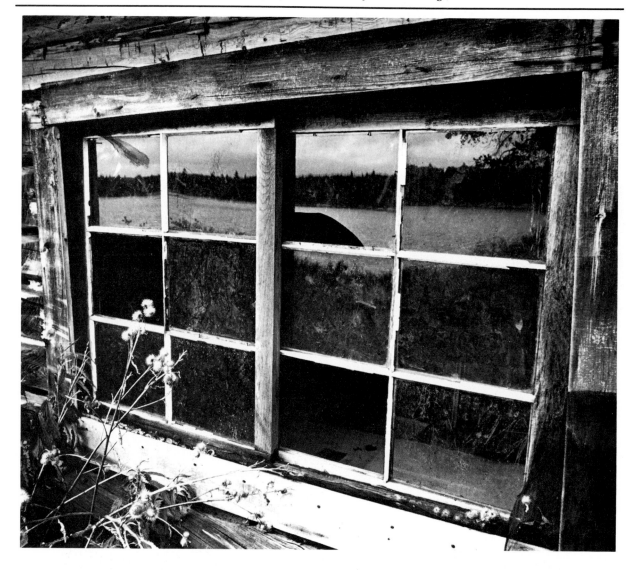

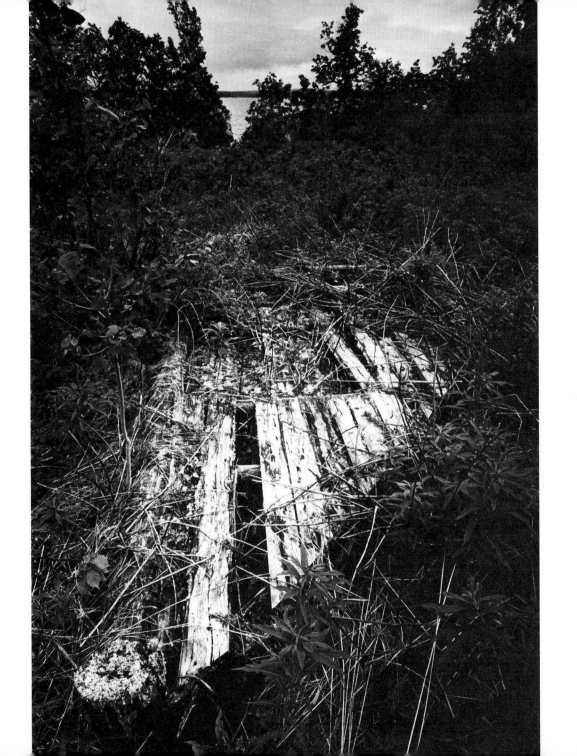

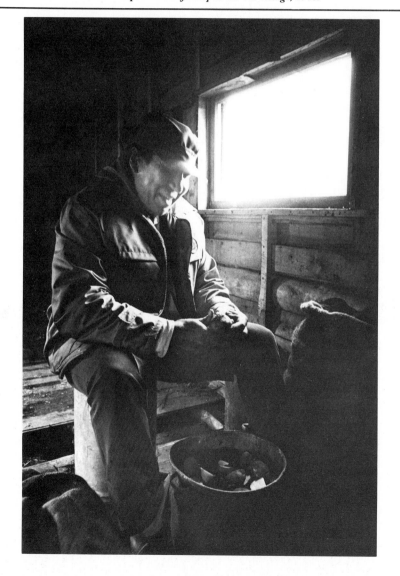

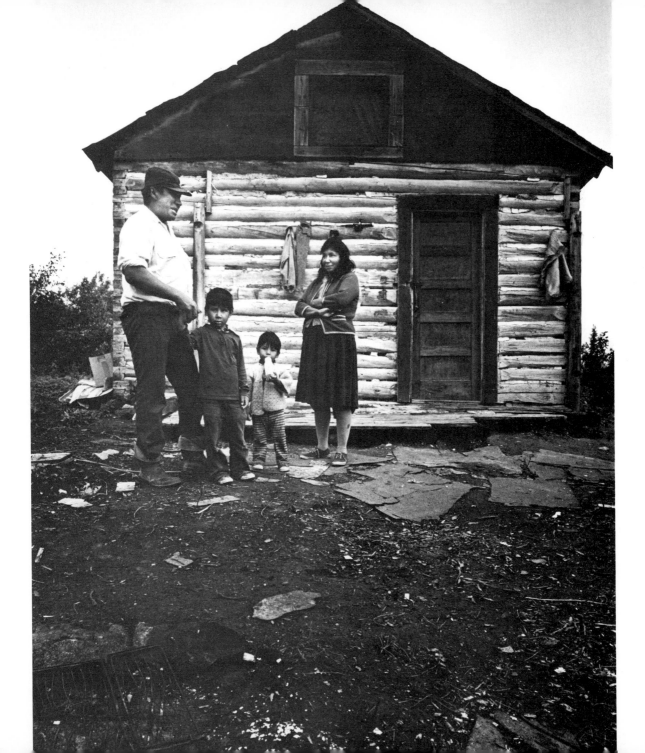

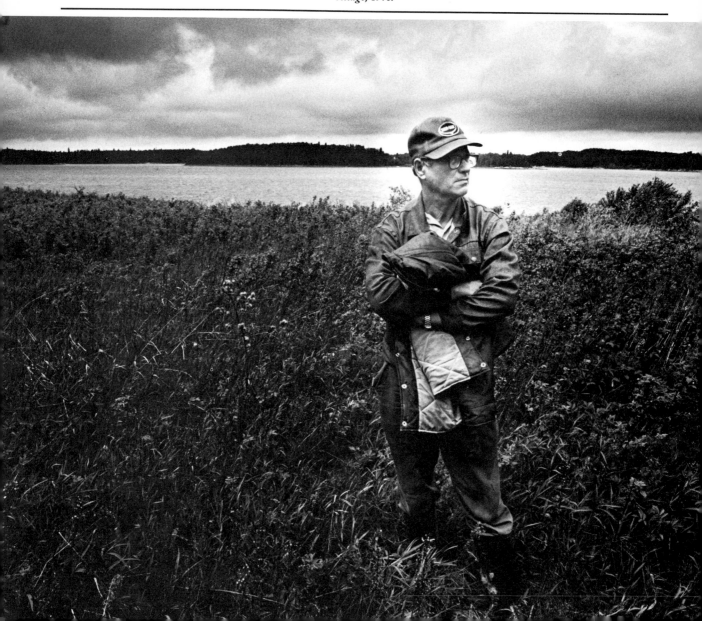

Andy Keewatin on the site of his former home at the old village, 1976.

the trap lines in winter, sometimes taking two or three of his seven children with him. But in summer, with the fishing gone, there wasn't much left to do, for children or their parents.

"I used to go out once a month on a drunk. But not every day, like you see now. I don't like their way of life. I hate to say it, but . . . I didn't want my kids involved in that kind of life. Right now, they are having three square meals a day, and that's my aim. I want to keep them that way for a little while longer yet."

In the spring of 1976, Gabe moved back to the old village with his wife Elizabeth and the children, repaired a decaying cabin and began his work in the garden. Gabe's move was part of an experiment by the band council to replace lost jobs and supplement costly food stocks. He was like a phantom in a ghost town, stepping back into the past to find solutions to present problems.

Grass was growing high, untended, at the old village. And many of the log homes that had housed the community for a century or more had fallen to the ground. The treaty house was a shell and the Roman Catholic church was almost hidden by underbrush, its roof, under which the Ojibways once prayed, full of gaping holes.

"Funny," commented Andy Keewatin, the former chief, as he toured the remains, "you leave something and it starts to deteriorate."

Andy remembered building the treaty house. He was twenty-one at the time and the people of Grassy Narrows were independent. "The government didn't put a cent into it," he said with pride. "It was built by the people themselves."

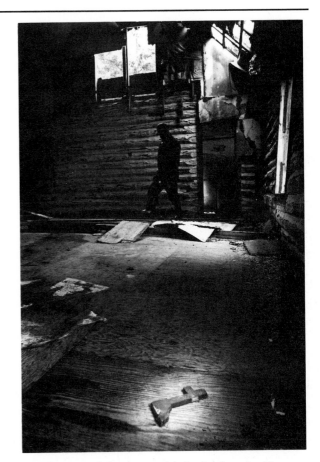

Time has ravaged the Roman Catholic church at the old village, 1976.

It was good here....
We have lost control.
Andy Keewatin

"It was good here. We were working for our-selves. We had our own gardens. That kept us occupied. The whole family worked together. Even the kids worked. The kids today don't know what it was like. Back here, they were part of the family. They played together once in a while. But they had to go home before dark. We had better control here. We have lost control.

"I can't make a garden where we live now. My boys, before they left me, we tried a little garden. But one time we were out and when we came back, there was nothing left of it. There are too many kids around.

"The people didn't want to live so close together. They wanted to be spread around. At the old village, a lot of people had their own clearings, like their own camp spots. They built their own homes. They surveyed their own places. But where we live now, Indian Affairs said we would have to live in one area on account of the school, and to get the hydro in and the water system. It sounded like a good idea at the time, but we shouldn't have had to move. They could have built the road in. We still could be living here."

Andy pondered the costs to his people as he rummaged through the remains of his early home-stead, flipping over a rusted chunk of kitchen stove with his boot. Memories of victims of these times flashed in his mind and he scanned the English River country, the island where the vacant Hudson's Bay store still stood, the clusters of aging log cabins, greying reminders of times when youngsters like Patrick Fobister lived lives free of tragedy.

"People, when they lived here, were proud of this place," said the former chief. "This was their own work. Now, they don't care where they live."

This was the place of Grassy's past, where, per-haps, answers might be found for the future. Here were traces of a happier existence and here were the graves of their ancestors, simple people whose uncomplicated lives followed the faithful patterns of the seasons, not the whims of industry, people who died before having to forsake their natural ways for the complex life style of the white man.

Graveyards dotted the old village, scattered in family plots. Some occupied peaceful plains, others ridges overlooking the troubled waters of Grassy Narrows. All were overgrown, obscured reminders of a happier past.

Andy searched for one of the forgotten burial grounds like a man intensely pursuing a memory that had seized his mind. He struggled through the underbrush, breaking his way through hip-deep bushes while branches whipped at his head. He plodded as though compelled to locate the graves — as though in finding them he might find answers.

"They used to be right along this ridge," he said, sweeping the overhanging branches aside as he reached the top. "Yes," he said, catching a glimpse of a white cross. "There is one."

A grave marker at the old village cemetery.

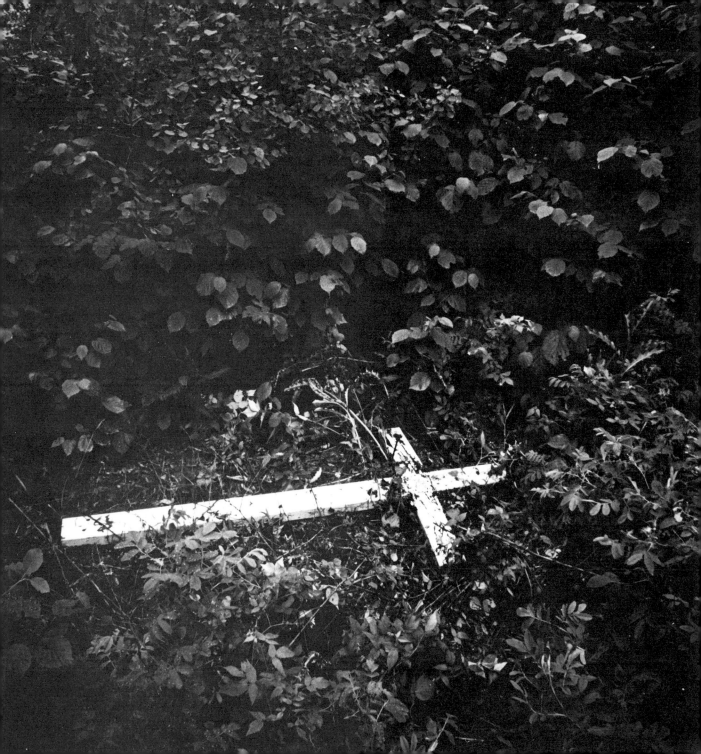

Epilogue

There are similarities between the plight of Grassy Narrows and the troubles facing many isolated native communities in North America. If anything, a sense of helplessness, victimization and frustration provides a common bond among Indians and Innuit, who believe they are being sacrificed in the name of "progress". However, events and politicians have so severely and arbitrarily worked against the people of Grassy over the last fifteen years that they have become much more than a stereotyped example of Indians in culture shock. All of the ingredients — conflicting pressures and vested interests — are here to be studied by other minority groups now under the pressure and threat of modern development, and by politicians and businessmen charged with the responsibility for guiding that development.

At Grassy, events have tragically demonstrated how history repeats itself despite the lessons of the past. With frightening predictability, decisions have been made outside the peoples' sphere of influence and imposed upon them, creating enormous social problems which seem to intensify with the passage of time. The toll can be counted in the graveyards of Grassy.

The lesson is not being lost on Ojibway and Cree leaders to the north in the area covered by Treaty Nine, where Reed Paper Company hopes to extend logging operations, provide more jobs and make more money from resource exploitation. The vow of Treaty Nine President Andrew Rickard to lay down his life rather than lose the forest is not without cause. History, rather than white pledges that consultation will produce safeguards, is shaping Indian response. In the case of Grassy, the people can only hope conditions will improve. They could hardly get much worse.

The future is not without promise, despite past disappointments. In 1977, Frank Miller replaced Leo Bernier as Ontario's minister of natural resources, politicians in Ottawa and Toronto were at least talking about joint redevelopment programs and Reed was making gestures that it wanted to help. Co-operation and good faith are long overdue. In addition, Premier William Davis finally yielded to public and private pressure to give Reed's expansion plans a thorough examination. He appointed Mr. Justice Patrick Hartt of the Supreme Court of Ontario to conduct an inquiry into the whole question of the impact of development on the north. The inquiry could take years and will likely follow the format set by British Columbia jurist, Thomas Berger, during his investigation of the Mackenzie Valley pipeline proposals. The Hartt inquiry should awaken politicians to the problems faced by the Indians and test the professed concern of elected representatives over spreading industrial pollution.

The people of Grassy, however, may be excused if they respond warily to oratory or overtures of assistance. Experience has been a brutal teacher. For fifteen years their dealings with white society have resulted in disrupted families and dead brothers. While mercury cannot as yet be diagnosed directly as the cause of any deaths, it has clearly worsened a dreadful situation and contributed to alcoholism and outbreaks of violence.

The origin of the troubles at Grassy can be found in the relocation program proposed and executed by the federal government in the first half of the 1960s. Consultation was minimal, and little effort was made to ease the wrenching transition from a wilderness to a modern existence. Lifestyles and languages were discarded almost overnight and ties with the past, the heritage of centuries, were frayed if not severed.

Life at the old village was not perfect; life seldom is. But what was lost was of value and the people who lived those days treasure their fading memories. Bill Fobister, for one, has vague recollections of elders such as Pierre Keesick and John Loon paddling the waters or snowshoeing over the frozen lakes with news from the outside world. There were pow wows and square dances at the Treaty House, and on Treaty Day in early summer, representatives of the Indian Affairs Department arrived with crisp new five-dollar bills to discharge the Crown's financial obligations to the first citizens. Treaty Day was often celebrated with a festival which lasted for days. Now, the people receive their treaty money by mail, or pick it up at the government office in Kenora.

"You don't see the pow wows any more," says Bill Fobister, whose three youngsters are more likely to remember fights and funerals than festivals. "Everything is changed. All of that is lost. I wish we could bring it back."

A rediscovery of past values and an appreciation of Ojibway culture must be found if the people of Grassy are to recover a sense of self-worth and community. Governments will have to accommodate this search. But government response seems to be predicated on the notion that the Indian must assimilate into white society or face the consequences. For the people of Grassy, the consequences have been enormous.

When mercury pollution undermined Grassy's fragile economy in the spring of 1970, even as the community was struggling to adjust to the relocation, Queen's Park showed little concern for the Indians' physical or financial well-being. Instead Queen's Park waited for Ottawa to respond. The administrations of premiers John Robarts and William Davis, through cabinet ministers George Kerr, Rene Brunelle and Leo Bernier, revealed an unwavering allegiance to industry. In the early days of the mercury crisis, the ministers denied that the pollution was extensive, dangerous and long lasting. When the pollution did not go away, the Ontario government and its federal counterpart allowed years to pass before undertaking a serious medical study of the downriver communities, and then only under the pressure of public opinion. The severity of the situation has consistently been downplayed and information suppressed.

To this day, the provincial and federal governments have no grip on the problem, no comprehensive program to compensate for the social and medical consequences of pollution, let alone effective pollution-control regulations. The government depends heavily on industry's good faith to meet whatever standards are set. These are often violated with impunity, since industry is expected to monitor its own waste discharges, and government inspection is inadequate.

Throughout this sorry episode, industry's role has been disappointing. Despite the acceptance of a moral and social responsibility by Reed Paper and its predecessor, Dryden Pulp and Paper Company, no representatives of the company have bothered to visit the affected communities, even as a gesture of concern. Only after a public outcry was raised over its expansion plans in the area of Treaty Nine did the company offer to meet with the senior governments to consider a program of assistance. Those talks have produced no proposal of substance.

Should the Indians seek a legal settlement of their grievances? After six years the provincial government's case against Dow Chemical is unresolved. Barney Lamm is no nearer settlement with Reed Paper than Queen's Park is with Dow. Among other defences, the Dryden company has stated that the waters of Ball Lake are not polluted — and if they are polluted the company is not responsible because, among other things, there are natural sources of mercury; moreover, according to the company, the waters of Ball Lake do not come from the Wabigoon. The company also denied that anything escaped from its plant, and if anything did escape, the company did not know it was harmful. In any case, says the company in its defence, the Lamms

closed their lodge voluntarily and were harmed by their own public statements.

Legal actions require that proof of liability be established, an exercise that can consume years, during which time the case becomes more difficult to reconstruct. Victims, meanwhile, continue to suffer hardship. The complexity of environmental pollution often seems to preclude just legal solutions. Victims must trace the contaminant to its sources, overcome arguments that background contamination is to blame, establish the extent of damage. Complicating the issue even further are government regulations governing the discharge of certain pollutants into the environment. Can a company which meets existing regulations be held legally responsible if discharges within the regulations eventually prove dangerous or harmful? In Japan, the court ruled that Chisso Corporation was liable despite compliance with legislation. It has yet to be seen whether a Canadian court would draw a similarly sweeping conclusion.

Legal and monetary solutions alone will not repair the damage done by mercury pollution at Grassy Narrows. The people of Grassy have already received significant material concessions from the provincial and federal governments — a community hall, day care centre, housing and the like. Grassy is not alone. Native communities across the country have been reaping financial benefits from a rising federal budget for Indian affairs, now about $500 million annually. If all this money were distributed among the Indians, it would represent an annual allotment of nearly $2,000 for each of the 275,000 status Indians and Innuits in Canada, or roughly $10,000 per family. This is exclusive of money paid out by federal and provincial departments under conventional programs such as family allowance and pensions. One official in Ottawa estimates government spending on Indians totals as much as $800 million a year, or about $12,500 a family. During World War II the government's budget was a pittance, an embarrassing $5 million. But despite the hundredfold increase in spending, social conditions have in many ways deteriorated in the clash of cultures. The investment of dollars has failed to return the desired human dividends. According to Indian leaders, this is primarily because bureaucracy strangles worthy programs, provides for only marginal participation by the people the programs are meant to serve, and leads to frustration.

The senior governments have belatedly attempted to stimulate self-sufficiency at Grassy Narrows, but they must recognize that industrial enterprise on the reserve will probably not make a profit. Business efforts such as the canoe factory, halting and uncertain, suggest that Grassy will forever be partly dependent on government handouts of one kind or another for economic survival. However, small industry should be encouraged; the people are anxious to break the welfare crutch and have meaningful work.

The economic base provided by guiding and commercial fishing must be replaced. It will undoubtedly cost more money than the $4.3-million program initially proposed by the camp operators in 1971, but the English-Wabigoon should be closed, the camps relocated and a system of transportation provided for Indian guides and commercial fishermen. If Reed Paper means what it says, it could send experienced business people to help industries on the reserve. Even at this late date, there is an urgent need for a committee of Indian leaders from Grassy and Whitedog, provincial and federal politicians and representatives of Reed Paper to chart a program of recovery.

Essential to any recovery effort is the support of the people of Grassy. They must be fully involved in the process and dictate its terms. Consultation must be real, not pretended, if a successful program is to be accomplished. "The lesson to be learned here," said school principal Dennis Clark, "is not to impose something from the outside, but to let the people who live here decide what they want. One of the assistant deputy ministers of Indian Affairs has said that we have to allow ourselves the luxury of letting the native people make their own mistakes. Maybe that's what has to be done."

It will not be easy. The years of turbulence at Grassy Narrows have created a leadership void. Five men have tried to serve as chief in the last three years, each surrendering to unpredictable shifts of opinion within the band or the sheer pressure of the job. The latest chief is young and the task enormous. Band officials have also come and gone with disturbing regularity, unable to cope with or resolve the tremendous problems confronting them.

Perhaps one of the benefits of this whole sorry affair will be a greater unity among the native groups in the region, and across the country, and an increased political awareness which can be mobilized to defend their interests from further erosion by outside forces.

Beyond the immediate problems facing Grassy, governments should be addressing themselves to the broader questions posed by the impact of industrial pollution on innocent victims. Existing legal remedies are too costly, too tedious and, ultimately, weighted in favor of the polluter. Once again, we can learn from the Japanese experience by passing stiffer laws and penalties to reduce industrial discharges and establishing an environmental compensation mechanism. Recognizing the need to avoid costly lawsuits and to relieve victims of the burden of proof, the Japanese in 1974 enacted a compensation law for the benefit of pollution victims. Funded by levies on industries, calculated on their environmental impact, the law provides medical care benefits and payments, handicap allowances and special compensation for survivors of deadly pollution such as Minamata Disease and for dependents of victims. In the case of Minamata Disease, only two symptoms need to be medically confirmed in order for a victim to qualify for benefits, administered by a review board. The governments in Canada possess detailed information on Japan's compensation program. They require only the will to act.

The people of Grassy Narrows have paid a heavy price for our material progress over the years. Introduction of such an act would demonstrate a new sense of responsibility on the part of government, and the people who elect it.

In a speech delivered in September, 1976, Prime Minister Pierre Trudeau chose to quote Indian Chief Seattle's warning that "whatever befalls the earth will befall the sons of the earth."

"And what is befalling the earth", Trudeau said, "is known to all of us. The high techniques, the high mechanistic civilization which we have developed has produced great abundance, great affluence, but it is also destroying the earth — destroying the rivers and the streams, fouling the air and the land, destroying the landscape. Even the mighty oceans are endangered. And as we know, when the oceans are dead, the planet will be dead."

Now it is time to decide how to stop the onslaught.